MW00337895

STUDENT WORKBOOK FOR

UNDERSTANDING
Medical
Surgical
Nursing

FIFTH EDITION

UNDERSTANDING
Medical
Surgical
Nursing

FIFTH EDITION

Paula D. Hopper, MSN, RN, CNE
Professor of Nursing
Jackson College
Jackson, Michigan

Linda S. Williams, MSN, RN
Professor of Nursing
Jackson College
Jackson, Michigan

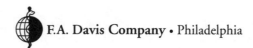
F.A. Davis Company • Philadelphia

F.A. Davis Company
1915 Arch Street
Philadelphia, PA 19103
www.fadavis.com

Copyright © 2015 by F.A. Davis Company

Copyright © 2015 by F.A. Davis Company. All rights reserved. This book is protected by copyright. No part of it may be reproduced, stored in a retrieval system, or transmitted in any form or by any means, electronic, mechanical, photocopying, recording, or otherwise, without written permission from the publisher.

Printed in the United States of America

Last digit indicates print number: 10 9 8 7 6 5 4 3 2 1

Acquisitions Editor: Lisa B. Houck
Director of Content Development: Darlene D. Pedersen
Content Project Manager: Elizabeth D. Hart
Illustration & Design Manager: Carolyn O'Brien

As new scientific information becomes available through basic and clinical research, recommended treatments and drug therapies undergo changes. The author(s) and publisher have done everything possible to make this book accurate, up to date, and in accord with accepted standards at the time of publication. The author(s), editors, and publisher are not responsible for errors or omissions or for consequences from application of the book, and make no warranty, expressed or implied, in regard to the contents of the book. Any practice described in this book should be applied by the reader in accordance with professional standards of care used in regard to the unique circumstances that may apply in each situation. The reader is advised always to check product information (package inserts) for changes and new information regarding dose and contraindications before administering any drug. Caution is especially urged when using new or infrequently ordered drugs.

ISBN 13: 978-0-8036-4069-6

Authorization to photocopy items for internal or personal use, or the internal or personal use of specific clients, is granted by F.A. Davis Company for users registered with the Copyright Clearance Center (CCC) Transactional Reporting Service, provided that the fee of $.25 per copy is paid directly to CCC, 222 Rosewood Drive, Danvers, MA 01923. For those organizations that have been granted a photocopy license by CCC, a separate system of payment has been arranged. The fee code for users of the Transactional Reporting Service is: 8036-4069-6/11 0 + $.25.

NOTE TO THE STUDENT

The *Student Workbook for Understanding Medical Surgical Nursing* has been written and edited by the authors to accompany the fifth edition of *Understanding Medical Surgical Nursing*. We have included exercises that not only help you review content, but also will help you develop your critical thinking abilities. It is essential for you to be able to think critically about the content as you prepare for the NCLEX-PN. We hope you will use this resource as well as your electronic study guide and the great resources on Davis*Plus*.

SUGGESTIONS FOR USING THE STUDY GUIDE

Checklists for Learning Success are provided at the beginning of each unit. You can use these checklists to track your study of the major topics.

Each chapter includes:

- An exercise to help you practice chapter vocabulary items. It is important to understand the underlying vocabulary before attempting to apply the terms to understand the remainder of the information in each chapter.
- Basic matching, true/false, word scramble, and other exercises to allow you to practice and understand medical-surgical nursing information. These exercises are most helpful for developing knowledge and recall of material.
- Critical thinking exercises to help you practice your new knowledge in patient situations and make good clinical judgments. We feel strongly that you must learn to think critically, rather than just memorize facts. The answers we provide for the critical thinking exercises are just some of the possibilities. You will come up with additional answers of your own as your knowledge base expands.
- NCLEX-PN style questions to provide practice in applying your new knowledge. Rationale for why an answer is correct or incorrect has been included to strengthen your critical thinking and test-taking abilities.
- Function and Assessment chapters also include a labeling exercise to help you review basic anatomy.

STUDY GUIDE ANSWERS

- To students: Study Guide answers are posted on the instructor's Davis*Plus* site. Ask your instructor about accessing answers.
- To instructors: Study Guide answers are posted on the instructor's Davis*Plus* site. Students do not have access to Study Guide answers. Please provide answers to students according to your needs.

We hope you find this study guide useful. Happy studying!

PAULA D. HOPPER AND LINDA S. WILLIAMS

Contents

unit ONE

Understanding Health Care Issues

CHECKLIST FOR LEARNING SUCCESS

Critical Thinking	Evidence-Based Practice	Issues	Cultural Influences	Alternative/Complementary
❏ Critical thinking traits	❏ Evidence-based practice	❏ Health care delivery	❏ Cultural diversity	❏ Alternative versus
❏ Knowledge base	❏ Use of evidence-based	❏ Economic issues	❏ Communication	complementary therapies
❏ Critical thinking skills	practice	❏ Nursing/health team	❏ Space	❏ Allopathic/Western medicine
❏ Problem solving	❏ Identifying evidence	❏ Leadership in nursing	❏ Time orientation	❏ Ayurveda
❏ Role of the LPN/LVN	❏ Evidence-based practice	practice	❏ Social organization	❏ Chinese medicine
❏ Nursing process	process	❏ Career opportunities	❏ Environmental control	❏ Chiropractic
❏ Data collection	❏ Six steps of evidence-	❏ Ethics and values	❏ Health care providers	❏ Homeopathy
❏ Documentation of data	based practice	❏ Ethical obligations and	❏ Biological variations	❏ Naturopathy
❏ Nursing diagnosis	❏ Evidence-based practice,	nursing	❏ Death and dying	❏ American Indian medicine
❏ Planning care	quality and safety	❏ Nursing code of ethics	❏ Cultural groups	❏ Osteopathy
❏ Prioritizing care	❏ Quality and Safety	❏ Building blocks of ethics	❏ Culturally competent care	❏ Herbal therapy
❏ Identifying interventions	Education for Nurses	❏ Ethical theories		❏ Relaxation therapies
❏ Implementation	(QSEN) project	❏ Ethical decision making		❏ Massage therapy
❏ Evaluation	❏ Joint Commission's 2014	❏ Legal concepts		❏ Aquatherapy
	National Patient Safety	❏ HIPAA		❏ Heat and cold
	Goals	❏ Nursing liability and the law		❏ Safety/effectiveness
				❏ Role of LPN/LVN

1

Critical Thinking and the Nursing Process

VOCABULARY

Define the following terms and use them in sentences.

Nursing process

Definition: _____

Sentence: _____

Critical thinking

Definition: _____

Sentence: _____

Assessment

Definition: _____

Sentence: _____

Objective data

Definition: _____

Sentence: _____

Subjective data

Definition: _____

Sentence: _____

Nursing diagnosis

Definition: _____

Sentence: _____

Evaluation

Definition: _____

Sentence: _____

Vigilance

Definition: _____

Sentence: _____

SUBJECTIVE AND OBJECTIVE DATA

Identify the following data as subjective (symptom) or objective (sign).

1. Pain _____

2. Shortness of breath _____

3. Edema (swelling) _____

4. Capillary refill 2 seconds _____

5. Nausea _____

6. Vomiting _____

7. Dizziness _____

8. Cyanosis _____

9. Numbness _____

10. Indigestion _____

11. Pale _____

12. Serum potassium 3.6 mEq/L _____

13. Palpitations (feeling of racing heart) _____

14. Blood pressure 130/82 mm Hg _____

15. White blood cell count 7000/mm^3 _____

CRITICAL THINKING

Sometimes cognitive maps are used to organize thinking. Look at samples in any of the Function and Assessment chapters under Aging Changes. Some of the workbook chapters will ask you to make a cognitive map, so here is an opportunity to practice. Consider a time when you have had a headache or other discomfort. Fill in the spaces with information related to the WHAT'S UP? questions. See Chapter 1 Answers for one patient's responses. Once you have the questions answered, you could go even further and make links with possible interventions. There is no one right way to make a cognitive map—use your imagination!

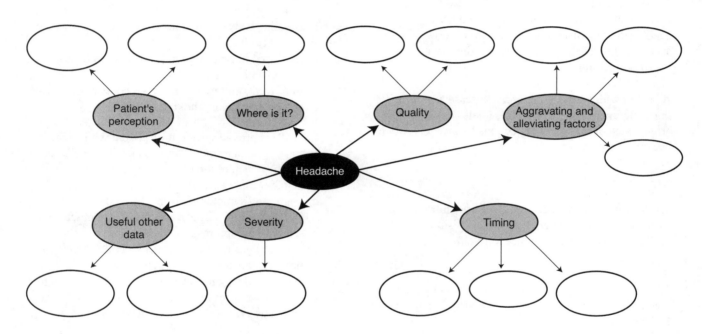

REVIEW QUESTIONS—CONTENT REVIEW

Choose the best answer unless directed otherwise.

1. Which one of the following is a nursing diagnosis?
   1. Peptic ulcer
   2. Pneumonia
   3. Ineffective airway clearance
   4. Myocardial infarction

2. Which one of the following is a medical diagnosis?
   1. Hiatal hernia
   2. Impaired mobility
   3. Powerlessness
   4. Anxiety

3. An LPN wishes to learn why a patient's lung sounds have crackles and questions the physician during morning rounds. Which critical thinking attitude is the nurse exhibiting?
   1. Intellectual humility
   2. Intellectual sense of justice
   3. Intellectual empathy
   4. Intellectual integrity

4. The LVN is caring for a patient with diabetes. In what order should the nurse carry out the nursing process? Place all steps in correct sequential order.
   1. Implement plan of care
   2. Assist with evaluation
   3. Collect data
   4. Assist with development of nursing diagnoses
   5. Assist with planning of outcomes and interventions

5. Which of the following statements best defines *critical thinking*?
   1. Orderly, goal-directed thinking
   2. Clear thinking during critical situations
   3. Constructive feedback about nursing actions
   4. Critical evaluation of patient responses to care

REVIEW QUESTIONS—TEST PREPARATION

Choose the best answer unless directed otherwise.

6. The LPN is reviewing the nursing care plan for a patient with acute pain related to a fractured ankle. Which of the following would determine whether the care plan is effective?
   1. Assessment of the patient's ability to walk
   2. Evaluation of the patient's fracture on X-ray
   3. Elevating the patient's foot on two pillows
   4. Evaluation of the patient's pain rating on a 10-point scale.

7. A patient with a history of cardiac disease reports a feeling of tightness in the chest that radiates down the left arm. Which of the following actions by the LPN should be carried out immediately?
   1. Check the patient's vital signs.
   2. Formulate nursing diagnoses related to an acute myocardial infarction.
   3. Determine the patient's outcome after nitroglycerin has been administered.
   4. Plan interventions to reduce long-term cardiac damage.

8. The LPN is documenting patient data. Which of the following should the nurse document under objective data?
   1. Denies nausea
   2. Shortness of breath
   3. Heart rate 72 beats per minute
   4. Midsternal chest pain

9. A patient is admitted with chest pain, which has resolved. The patient states, "I hope I can live a normal life." According to Maslow's hierarchy of needs, which of the following levels is best reflected by this statement?
   1. Physiological needs
   2. Safety and security
   3. Love and belonging
   4. Self-esteem

10. A patient has a nursing diagnosis of impaired swallowing related to muscle weakness as evidenced by drooling, coughing, and choking. Which of the following outcomes is appropriate for this patient's nursing diagnosis?
    1. Improved airway clearance within 8 hours as evidenced by clear lung sounds and productive cough
    2. Baseline body weight maintained as evidenced by no weight loss
    3. Improved muscle strength as evidenced by ability to sit up while eating
    4. Improved swallowing within 48 hours as evidenced by no coughing or choking

11. The LPN is providing care for a patient with a medical diagnosis of congestive heart failure who is very short of breath. Which of the following is a nursing diagnosis that is correctly stated in the PES (problem, etiology, and signs and symptoms) format?
    1. Deficient knowledge related to disease process and self-care for shortness of breath
    2. Impaired gas exchange related to excess interstitial fluid as evidenced by respiratory rate of 32 per minute and patient stating he feels short of breath
    3. Congestive heart failure related to decreased cardiac output as evidenced by abnormal arterial blood gasses
    4. Acute dyspnea related to congestive heart failure as evidenced by swollen lower extremities and confusion.

Evidence-Based Practice

2

VOCABULARY

Define the following terms.

1. Evidence-based practice

_____

2. Randomized controlled trials

_____

3. Research

_____

4. Systematic review

_____

EVIDENCE-BASED PRACTICE

1. Evidence is the _____ of effectiveness behind nursing practice.

2. It is important for the _____ in which the evidence will be used to be considered.

3. Evidence-based practice (EBP) is a complex but important, necessary process to facilitate _____ care and optimal patient outcomes.

4. Evidence-based practice is used by nurses to give the best _____ possible.

5. Level I is the _____ evidence and is an analysis of many _____ controlled trials.

6. Nurses will know from measured _____ that they are giving the best care possible.

7. Evidence-based practice is considered the _____ standard of health care.

8. The Quality and Safety Education for Nurses (QSEN) project focuses on _____ education that promotes the continual improvement of quality and safety in patient care.

9. Patient-centered care meets the _____ needs and preferred schedules.

10. Evidence is the core _____ that directs safe, quality-driven, excellent patient care.

CRITICAL THINKING

Read the following case study and answer the questions.

Nurses on a surgical unit were interested in knowing if music would reduce the preoperative anxiety of patients on their unit.

1. How are these nurses contributing to quality care?

   _____

   _____

2. What should the nurses do to begin the process?

   _____

   _____

3. What are some examples of resources that can be used to find evidence? _____

   _____

4. The nurses found Level I research studies that showed music therapy could be beneficial in reducing anxiety. What step should the nurses take next?

_____

_____

5. The planned intervention was implemented, data were collected during the implementation, and now the pilot study has ended. What step should the nurses take next?

_____

_____

REVIEW QUESTIONS—CONTENT REVIEW

Choose the best answer unless directed otherwise.

1. Which of the following is considered significant evidence to guide nursing care?
   1. Research studies that are quasi-experimental
   2. Cochrane Reviews
   3. Nursing information from the Internet
   4. The opinion of a nationally known nursing expert

2. A nurse would like to find other studies on wound care that might be relevant to how wound care is done. Which of the following would be the best for searching for nursing articles on wound care?
   1. CINAHL
   2. Medline
   3. Cochrane Review
   4. PubMed

3. A nurse on the safety committee is assigned to review the current National Patient Safety Goals. In which of these ways will the nurse find the goals?
   1. Review Joanna Briggs Best Practices.
   2. Review a fundamentals nursing textbook.
   3. Go to www.jointcommission.org.
   4. Search Cochrane Reviews.

4. Which of the following best describes a randomized clinical trial (RCT)?
   1. An observational study designed to collect subjective data
   2. An experimental study in which multiple factors affecting the results are controlled
   3. A specific design categorizing modifiable and nonmodifiable risk factors
   4. Tracking of disease occurrence over a set period of time

5. Evidence-based practice most often begins with which of the following?
   1. Asking how to solve a clinical problem
   2. Initiating a literature search
   3. Analyzing available evidence
   4. Measuring baseline outcomes

REVIEW QUESTIONS—TEST PREPARATION

Choose the best answer unless directed otherwise.

6. The nurse is reviewing the patient's plan of care and ordered treatments. Which of the following is an independent nursing intervention? **Select all that apply.**
   1. Giving Tylenol 650 milligrams orally every 4 hours as needed (prn)
   2. Assisting patient to position of comfort
   3. Giving hand massage daily
   4. Initiating high-risk fall protocol
   5. Placing call button within reach at all times
   6. Teaching deep breathing and relaxation techniques as needed

7. A nurse on the research committee is assigned to review the best evidence on patient centered bathing. Which of the following kinds of evidence would the nurse select for Level I research? **Select all that apply.**
   1. A Cochrane review
   2. One RCT
   3. Four quasi-experimental studies that show similar results
   4. The opinion of a national nursing expert on the subject
   5. A Joanna Briggs Best Practice Review

8. The nurse will include which of the following in applying the process of evidence-based practice to patient centered care? **Select all that apply.**
   1. Evaluate the change.
   2. Determine current practice.
   3. Ask a burning question.
   4. Know how to conduct an RCT.
   5. Search for the best available evidence.
   6. Make it happen.

9. The nurse provides care for residents on an Alzheimer's unit and is working with family members of a 67-year-old patient who was recently admitted. Which of the following statements reveals the nurse's awareness of evidence-based reality orientation practice?
   1. "Patients on this unit are generally very sweet, so your loved one will quickly fit right in."
   2. "Our dietician provides high-protein snacks twice daily to help prevent brain degeneration."
   3. "You'll notice clocks, calendars, and the use of patient pictures in the hallways to help residents stay oriented."
   4. "Alzheimer's is a devastating disease, so it is mandatory that family members participate in our weekly support groups."

10. A nurse investigating the effect of 12-hour shifts on medication errors identifies 962 articles published on the topic of 12-hour shifts in the past 5 years. Which action should the nurse take next?
    1. Find out how many of the articles can be found at the institution.
    2. Request all 962 articles and determine their validity.
    3. Limit the request to articles published in the past 3 years.
    4. Narrow the search to identify which articles discuss medication errors.

Issues in Nursing Practice

VOCABULARY

Match the term with the appropriate definition or statement.

1. _____ Assault
2. _____ Battery
3. _____ Defamation
4. _____ False imprisonment
5. _____ Outrage
6. _____ Invasion of privacy and wrongful disclosure of confidential information

1. Unlawful touching of another
2. Unlawful conduct that places another in the immediate fear of unlawful touching or battery; the real threat of bodily harm
3. Unlawful restriction of a person's freedom
4. Extreme and outrageous conduct by a defendant relating to the care of the patient or the body of a deceased individual
5. Wrongful injury to another's reputation or standing in a community; may be written (libel) or spoken (slander)
6. Liability when a patient's privacy is invaded physically or if records are released without authority

NURSING PRACTICE AND ETHICAL AND LEGAL PRINCIPLES

1. The health–illness continuum represents the potential shifting between _____ health and poor health throughout the _____ span.
2. Nurses must be _____ licensed to practice to _____ the public and maintain the _____ of health care services.
3. _____ is a central virtue in nursing.
4. Nursing care uses the following principles: ensuring _____ and respect, _____ confidentiality, respecting the patient's right to make care choices, and maintaining a professional relationship with the patient.
5. Effective leaders are _____ about the management process, _____, positive thinkers, and use _____ to earn the _____ of their coworkers.

VALUES CLARIFICATION

Complete the following sentences.

1. The one thing I have always wanted to do is

   _____.

2. If I inherited 5 million dollars, I would

   _____.

3. As president of the United States, I would

   _____.

4. If I died today, I would like my obituary to say

   _____.

5. If I could control the world and its destiny, I would

   _____.

Complete this list of things people value with any other items you believe should be included, then rank the value you believe each item has, with 1 being the highest value.

Rank	Valued Item	Rank	Valued Item
_____	Family	_____	Professionalism
_____	Career	_____	_____
_____	Religion	_____	_____
_____	Honor	_____	_____
_____	Material possessions	_____	_____
_____	Health	_____	_____
_____	Recreation	_____	_____

What have you learned about yourself by doing this exercise? What do the rankings signify? Can you identify yourself as more utilitarian or more deontological? (There are no answers to this section because this is an exercise requiring personal responses.)

CRITICAL THINKING

Read the following case study and answer the questions.

Mrs. Reo, a 5 foot, 3 inch, 105-lb, 86-year-old retired cleaning lady, was admitted to a general medical-surgical unit in a small rural hospital. She was diagnosed 3 months ago with metastatic cancer that had spread from her liver to her lungs and bone marrow. She received chemotherapy and radiation therapy for several weeks, but the treatment was not effective. She was admitted to the hospital because she became too weak to walk or care for herself at home. The cancer returned, and the large doses of oral narcotic medications taken at home were having little effect on her pain while increasing her confusion and weakness.

Her oncologist decided that further chemotherapy or radiation therapy would not be effective, and she ordered Mrs. Reo to be kept comfortable with medications. A continuous morphine intravenous (IV) drip was started to help control the pain. Even with this medication, Mrs. Reo cried out in pain, particularly when morning care was given, and begged the nurses not to move her. Because she was severely underweight, the skin over her bony prominences quickly became reddened and showed the beginning signs of breakdown.

The hospital standards of care for immobile patients require that they be repositioned at least every 2 hours. Mrs. Reo yelled so loudly when she was turned that the nursing staff wondered if they were really helping her or hurting her.

To help decide what should be done, the nurses who gave care to Mrs. Reo called a patient care conference. The manager of the unit stated clearly that the hospital standards of care required Mrs. Reo be repositioned at least every 2 hours to prevent skin breakdown, infections, and

perhaps sepsis. In her already weakened condition, an infection or sepsis would most likely be fatal. Betsy, who had been a licensed practical nurse for some 15 years, disagreed with the manager. Her feeling was that causing this obviously terminal patient so much pain by turning her was cruel and violated her dignity as a human being. She stated that she could not stand to hear Mrs. Reo yell anymore and refused to take care of her until some other decision was made about her nursing care. Sally, a new graduate nurse, felt that the patient should have some say in her own care and that perhaps some type of compromise could be reached about turning her, perhaps turning her less frequently or providing more pain relief medication. Monica, a registered nurse who had worked on the unit for 2 years, felt that the physician should make the decision about turning this patient, and then the nurses should follow the order. This last suggestion was met with strong negative comments by the other nurses present. They felt that patient comfort and turning were nursing measures.

1. What are the important ethical principles in this dilemma?

_____

_____

2. How does the Code of Ethics apply to this situation?

_____

_____

3. What are the legal issues?

_____

_____

4. Are there ever any situations when a nurse might legally and ethically violate a standard of care?

_____

_____

5. What are some other possible solutions to this dilemma? What types of consequences might they have?

_____

_____

(There are no correct answers to this section because this is an ethical exercise that has many choices to be considered for the best outcome for the patient. Discuss your options with classmates.)

REVIEW QUESTIONS—CONTENT REVIEW

Choose the best answer unless directed otherwise.

1. The ethical principle that the primary goal of health care and nursing is to do good for others is called which of the following?
   1. Autonomy
   2. Fidelity
   3. Beneficence
   4. Veracity

2. The ethical principle of nonmaleficence is defined as which of the following?
   1. Health care workers avoiding harm to patients
   2. Telling the truth to patients in all matters
   3. Being faithful to commitments made to patients
   4. The right of self-determination of patients

3. Which of the following is the term used to describe an ethical situation that arises in which there is a choice between two equally unfavorable alternatives?
   1. Tort
   2. Ethical antagonism
   3. Contraindication
   4. Ethical dilemma

4. Which of the following is the first step in the ethical decision-making process?
   1. Analyze the alternatives.
   2. Identify the ethical dilemma.
   3. Consider the consequences of the actions.
   4. Make a decision.

5. Ethical dilemmas most often involve which of the following situations?
   1. A conflict of basic human rights
   2. Violations of the Nurses' Code of Ethics
   3. Nurses who do not understand the ethical code
   4. Patients who wish to die

6. When applying the ethical principle of autonomy to patient care, the nurse should understand that which of the following is applicable to autonomy?
   1. Autonomy is an absolute principle that has no exceptions.
   2. Only patients who are awake and oriented have the right to autonomy.
   3. Under certain conditions, autonomy can be limited.
   4. Autonomy is the same as the principle of nonmaleficence.

7. Which of the following punishments distinguishes criminal liability from civil liability?
   1. Personal liability
   2. Financial recovery
   3. Loss of license
   4. Potential loss of freedom

8. Which of the following is an unintentional tort?
   1. Negligence
   2. Outrage
   3. Assault
   4. Privacy invasion

REVIEW QUESTIONS—TEST PREPARATION

Choose the best answer unless directed otherwise.

9. A patient with emphysema is being seen by the home health nurse. The patient is on oxygen, lives alone, and is able to perform activities of daily living, prepare meals, and do light household tasks with rest periods. The patient is unable to perform yard work, which was a favorite hobby. Which of the following would describe the patient's location on the health–illness continuum?
   1. Near death
   2. High-level wellness
   3. Poor health
   4. Moderate-level wellness

10. A Nurses' Code of Ethics states, "The nurse safeguards the patient's right to privacy by judiciously protecting information of a confidential nature." This statement is based on which of the following principles?
    1. The right to privacy is an inalienable right of all persons.
    2. The nurse–patient relationship is based on trust.
    3. A breach of confidentiality may expose the nurse to liability.
    4. Nurses know what is best for patients' health care.

11. A patient asks the nurse what is the purpose of a new medication. The nurse responds, "The medication will help you feel better, and not to worry about it." The nurse's response demonstrates which of the following conditions?
    1. Therapeutic communication
    2. Paternalism
    3. Lack of knowledge
    4. Legal obligations

12. The nurse attempts to apply the standard of best interest to a patient who has had a cardiac arrest and is now unconscious. Which of the following conditions is the most important factor for the nurse to consider?
    1. The patient's wishes as expressed before becoming unconscious
    2. The family's wishes now that the patient can no longer communicate
    3. The patient's chances for survival after the cardiac arrest
    4. The physician's orders regarding future arrest situations

13. The LVN is considering whether the task of taking a blood pressure on a 78-year-old resident with hypertension can be delegated to a nursing assistant. Which of the following steps should the nurse consider in this decision-making process for delegation? **Select all that apply.**
    1. Right task
    2. Right circumstances
    3. Right patient
    4. Right communication
    5. Right supervision
    6. Right route

4

Cultural Influences on Nursing Care

VOCABULARY

Match the term with the appropriate definition or statement.

1. _____ Belief
2. _____ Cultural awareness
3. _____ Cultural competence
4. _____ Ethnic
5. _____ Ethnocentrism
6. _____ Generalization
7. _____ Stereotype
8. _____ Value
9. _____ Worldview
10. _____ Custom
11. _____ Cultural sensitivity
12. _____ Assimilation

1. A usual way of acting in a given situation
2. Accepted as true, need not be proven
3. Focuses on knowledge and appreciation of history and ancestry of other cultures
4. Avoiding actions that may offend another person's cultural beliefs
5. Belief that "my way is the only right way"
6. An assumption that needs validation
7. An opinion or belief about someone because of ethnic background
8. Belonging to a subgroup of a larger cultural group
9. Way a person perceives the world
10. The process of taking on a dominant culture's values, sometimes with risk of losing one's own cultural heritage
11. Using knowledge and skills about another culture to provide care
12. A principle or belief that has worth to an individual or group

CULTURAL CHARACTERISTICS

Answer the following questions. Discuss with a classmate.

1. What are some examples of primary characteristics of culture? _____

_____

_____

2. What are some examples of secondary characteristics of culture? _____

_____

_____

3. What is meant by traditional health care practitioners? Give an example. _____

_____

_____

4. What are some characteristics of people who are primarily present oriented? Past oriented? Future oriented?

_____

_____

_____

CRITICAL THINKING: IMMIGRANTS

There are no correct or incorrect answers to the following questions. Share your thoughts with your classmates.

1. Are immigrants taking away from the United States, or are they adding to its richness? Give specific examples, and share your reasons for your position.

_____

_____

_____

2. Identify health care difficulties that new immigrants must overcome in the United States. How might you, as a nurse, help them overcome these difficulties?

_____

_____

_____

(There are no answers to this section because this is an exercise requiring personal responses.)

CRITICAL THINKING: PERSONAL INSIGHTS

Answer the following questions. Consider how people from other cultures might answer differently.

1. What do you personally do to prevent illness?

_____

_____

_____

2. What home remedies do you use when you have a minor illness such as a cold or flu? Do you use over-the-counter medications to treat yourself? How might these over-the-counter medicines cause a problem with prescription medications?

_____

_____

_____

3. What significance does food have to you besides satisfying hunger?

_____

_____

_____

4. Are you usually on time for social events? For appointments? Why or why not?

_____

_____

_____

(There are no answers to this section because this is an exercise requiring personal responses.)

CRITICAL THINKING: BATHING

Read the following case study and answer the questions.

An older adult male Arab American patient refuses to be bathed by a female nurse's aide. He has not been bathed for 3 days, and today he really needs a bath. His family is at his bedside.

1. Why do you think he is refusing his bath?

_____

_____

_____

2. What alternatives do you have?

_____

_____

_____

3. What is the best solution to the problem?

_____

_____

_____

REVIEW QUESTIONS—CONTENT REVIEW

Choose the best answer unless directed otherwise.

1. Patients of Eastern European Jewish heritage who are getting married should be provided information on which disorder?
   1. Sickle cell anemia
   2. Thalassemia
   3. Lactose intolerance
   4. Tay-Sachs disease

2. A patient states, "I don't know why that foreign doctor needs to be here. I only want to see American doctors." This is an example of which of the following principles?
   1. Cultural sensitivity
   2. Cultural diversity
   3. Ethnocentrism
   4. Acculturation

3. Hispanic Americans and American Indians generally have a _____ (higher or lower) glucose level than whites.

REVIEW QUESTIONS—TEST PREPARATION

Choose the best answer unless directed otherwise.

4. A 26-year-old Pueblo American Indian mother arrives at the health clinic to receive treatment for a laceration on her leg. Accompanying her are her two children, who missed their immunization appointments last month because she did not have transportation. As the clinic nurse, what is the best approach to ensure that the children get their immunizations?
   1. Give the immunizations today.
   2. Reschedule the appointment for next month at the regular hours for the immunization clinic.
   3. Reschedule the immunizations for when she returns to have her stitches removed.
   4. Ask the community health nurse to go to the home to give the immunizations.

5. A Guatemalan patient died after a cardiac arrest. His wife is uncontrollably wailing and shouting "Vaya con dios!" and lying on the floor shaking. What action should the nurse take?
   1. Call a cardiac arrest team.
   2. Immediately call for a stretcher and get her off the floor.
   3. Calmly remain beside her and talk to her.
   4. Call the house physician to order a tranquilizer.

6. A Laotian child is brought to the emergency department by the school nurse. She wants the child examined for the possibility of child abuse because he has several circular ecchymotic areas 2 inches in diameter on his back. What action should the intake nurse perform?
   1. Call the child welfare authorities to intervene.
   2. Explain to the school nurse that the bruised areas may be caused by the traditional Chinese practice of cupping.
   3. Inform the child's mother that he is in the emergency department.
   4. Report the school nurse for not getting consent from the mother to bring the child to the emergency department.

7. A 42-year-old Arab American patient has chronic renal failure. He asks the nurse where he can purchase a kidney for transplantation. Which response is best?
   1. Organs cannot be purchased in the United States.
   2. Explain the ethical dilemma in purchasing organs.
   3. Call the unit supervisor.
   4. Give him the area organ procurement telephone number.

8. A 12-year-old child from a traditional Korean American family is newly diagnosed with diabetes mellitus. His home health nurse is to teach the patient and family diabetes care. Both parents and the child can administer his insulin and recite the signs and symptoms of hypoglycemia and hyperglycemia. They are highly educated and read and speak English well. Which is the best first step in teaching them about nutrition therapy for diabetes?
   1. Give them a food exchange list for a diabetic diet.
   2. Determine whether they can calculate calories in a sample meal.
   3. Assess current dietary food practices.
   4. Have them make an appointment with a consulting dietitian.

9. A 46-year-old Cuban American high school teacher has been admitted for cancer of the breast. She wants her religious counselor, a *santero,* to visit. Which action should the nurse take?
   1. Ask the nursing supervisor to see if a visit from a *santero* is permitted.
   2. Tell her that *santeros* are not permitted in the hospital.
   3. Suggest that she see a hospital priest instead.
   4. Tell her a visit is fine, but for safety reasons she should tell the nurse or physician before accepting any treatments.

10. A 62-year-old Hispanic Peruvian woman is in the operating room having bypass surgery. Eighteen family members arrive on the unit and wait in her room, which is shared by two other patients. Which is the best solution to this problem?
   1. Allow two family members to wait in the room and send the rest of them to the cafeteria.
   2. Send all of them to the lobby and tell them they will be notified when the patient returns to her room.
   3. Allow only her husband and mother to visit.
   4. Assign the patient to a private room and allow the family to wait there.

11. A 42-year-old African American patient is 40 pounds overweight. She admits to baking pies with lard and frying food in bacon grease, practices she does not wish to stop. To reduce fat and calories, what can the home health nurse encourage her to do?
   1. Do not purchase lard.
   2. Reduce the portion size when she cuts her pies.
   3. Bake two separate pies, one for her and one for her family.
   4. Continue baking with lard, but reduce calories she receives from other foods in her diet.

12. A 41-year-old Hispanic woman has had a mastectomy for cancer of the breast. Her physician recommends radiation therapy. She says, "What is the use? My life is in God's hands anyway." Which of the following responses is appropriate?
   1. Agree with her, but tell her she must accept the radiation or she will die.
   2. Ensure that she understands all of the implications of her decision before accepting it.
   3. Keep encouraging her to think about the radiation, and ask all of the other staff to do the same.
   4. Have her ask her physician to prescribe chemotherapy instead of radiation therapy.

13. A 72-year-old Iranian patient says he will not be able to take his morning antibiotic, which is scheduled every 8 hours, because he is celebrating Ramadan and has to fast from sunup to sundown. Which of the following actions should the nurse take?
   1. Explain that the medicine must be taken now to maintain the blood level of the drug.
   2. Rearrange his medication schedule so he can take all his medicines between sundown and sunup.
   3. Omit the medicine and record his refusal on the medication administration record.
   4. Ask his family to encourage him to take the medicine.

5

Complementary and Alternative Modalities

VOCABULARY

Match the term with the appropriate definition or statement.

1. _____ Alternative modality
2. _____ Complementary modality
3. _____ Homeopathy
4. _____ Naturopathy
5. _____ Ayurvedic
6. _____ Chiropractic

1. Illness is a result of falling out of balance with nature
2. Uses nutrition, herbs, and hydrotherapy
3. Illness is a result of nerve dysfunction
4. Added to a conventional therapy
5. Unconventional therapy
6. "Like cures like"

COMPLEMENTARY MODALITY: GUIDED IMAGERY

Describe the purpose of guided imagery. Write a teaching plan on how to do guided imagery. Try teaching it to a family member or friend.

Purpose: _____

_____

_____

Teaching Plan: _____

_____

_____

CRITICAL THINKING

Read the following case study and answer the questions.

Mrs. Lawless is admitted to your unit with heart failure and fluid overload. As you collect admission data, you find that she is taking feverfew, capsaicin, and St. John's Wort regularly in addition to her prescribed medications for heart failure. When you question her, she says that the salesperson at the health food store told her these herbs were safe to use with her other medications.

1. What is feverfew used for? _____

_____

2. What is capsaicin used for?

_____

_____

3. What is St. John's wort used for?

_____

_____

4. Where can you get information about the safety of taking these herbs with heart failure or with heart failure medications?

_____

_____

5. What should you tell Mrs. Lawless?

_____

_____

REVIEW QUESTIONS—CONTENT REVIEW

Choose the best answer unless directed otherwise.

1. Which of the following therapies would be considered a complementary modality?
   1. Using inhalers in addition to oral medications for asthma
   2. Participating in a cardiac rehabilitation program after having a heart attack
   3. Using echinacea instead of antibiotics for an upper respiratory infection
   4. Using progressive muscle relaxation in addition to muscle relaxants for back pain

2. Which of the following therapies would be considered an alternative modality?
   1. Using hydrotherapy in place of nonsteroidal anti-inflammatory drugs for arthritis
   2. Visiting a spiritual healer in addition to chemotherapy for cancer treatment
   3. Using antibiotics and bronchodilators for acute bronchitis
   4. Using aspirin for a headache

3. Which of the following terms describes traditional Western medicine?
   1. Homeopathy
   2. Naturopathy
   3. Allopathy
   4. Ayurveda

4. Which of the following herbal remedies is possibly effective against viruses and colds?
   1. Echinacea
   2. Feverfew
   3. Chamomile
   4. Ginger

5. The nurse recognizes which of the following as complementary or alternative therapies aimed at altering the body's energy? **Select all that apply.**
   1. Reiki
   2. Magnet therapy
   3. Music therapy
   4. Hydrotherapy
   5. Yoga
   6. Therapeutic touch

REVIEW QUESTIONS—TEST PREPARATION

Choose the best answer unless directed otherwise.

6. The nurse has provided instruction to a patient on how to use guided imagery. Which of the following statements by the patient would indicate to the nurse that further teaching is required?
   1. "I will focus on my breathing."
   2. "I imagine the ocean, including the smell, the sound, and the feel of the air."
   3. "I will relax all parts of my body."
   4. "I will keep my eyes open until the exercise is complete."

7. A patient tells a nurse that a chiropractor is going to do minor surgery to remove a small superficial lump on her neck. Which response by the nurse is best?
   1. "The lump is likely pressing against a nerve; that is why it needs to be removed."
   2. "You need to question your chiropractor's qualifications. Chiropractors do not perform surgery."
   3. "Chiropractors specialize in nerve function; removing the lump will restore normal nerve function."
   4. "Surgery might not be necessary; usually a simple chiropractic adjustment will relieve pressure on a nerve."

8. A patient admitted with chronic pain says he is interested in pursuing an alternative modality for his pain, but he is unsure how to determine whether it is safe. Which of the following responses by the nurse is best?
   1. "As long as the therapy does not include medication, it should be safe."
   2. "You should talk with your primary care practitioner before trying anything new."
   3. "Be careful, because many alternative therapies have dangerous side effects."
   4. "Traditional analgesics are always the safest treatment for chronic pain."

9. A nurse is interested in providing therapeutic touch therapy for her home care patient with severe pain. This will be her first experience with therapeutic touch. Which of the following steps is least appropriate before beginning to provide this new service?
   1. Obtain permission from the patient's physician and home care agency.
   2. Take classes on how to administer therapeutic touch.
   3. Tell the patient he will be able to reduce the number of medications he takes.
   4. Read current research on the use of therapeutic touch.

10. A patient is preparing to go home from the hospital after an anterior wall myocardial infarction. He has new prescriptions for isosorbide (Imdur), warfarin (Coumadin), atorvastatin (Lipitor), and aspirin. He also takes metformin (Glucophage) and glipizide (Glucotrol XL) for type 2 diabetes and takes self-prescribed ginseng daily. Which initial response by the nurse is best?
    1. "Ginseng can effectively lower blood glucose in patients with diabetes. It is a good choice for you."
    2. "Ginseng is a relatively safe herbal agent. Be sure to check out a reliable website for interactions before continuing to take it at home."
    3. "Ginseng, like other herbal agents, is unsafe to take with your prescribed medications."
    4. "I am concerned that ginseng could interact with your prescribed medications and affect your blood glucose and your blood clotting."

unit TWO

Understanding Health and Illness

CHECKLIST FOR LEARNING SUCCESS

Fluid, Electrolyte, and Acid–Base Balance and Imbalance	Nursing Care of Patients Receiving Intravenous (IV) Therapy	Nursing Care of Patients With Infections	Nursing Care of Patients in Shock	Nursing Care of Patients in Pain	Nursing Care of Patients With Cancer	Nursing Care of Patients Having Surgery	Nursing Care of Patients With Emergent Conditions and Disaster/ Bioterrorism Response
❑ Fluid balance	❑ Indications for IV therapy	❑ Infectious process	❑ Pathophysiology of shock	❑ Definitions of pain	❑ Review of normal anatomy and physiology	❑ Surgery urgency/ purpose	❑ Primary survey
❑ Dehydration	❑ Types of infusions	❑ Body's defense mechanisms	❑ Complications from shock	❑ Mechanism of pain transmission	❑ Pathophysiology and etiology	❑ Preoperative phase	❑ Secondary survey
❑ Fluid excess	❑ Methods of infusion	❑ Infectious disease	❑ Hypovolemic shock	❑ Types of pain	❑ Risk factors for cancer	❑ Preoperative assessment/ admission	❑ Shock
❑ Electrolyte balance	❑ Types of Fluids (tonicity)	❑ Community infection control	❑ Cardiogenic shock	❑ Nonopioid analgesics	❑ Cancer classification	❑ Nursing process:	❑ Anaphylaxis
❑ Sodium imbalances	❑ IV access	❑ Health care agency infection control	❑ Obstructive shock	❑ Opioid analgesics	❑ Early detection/ prevention	❑ Preoperative	❑ Major trauma
❑ Potassium imbalances	❑ Peripheral IV therapy	❑ Antibiotic-resistant infections	❑ Distributive shock	❑ Opioid antagonists	❑ Diagnostic tests	❑ Intraoperative phase	❑ Hypothermia
❑ Calcium imbalances	❑ Venipuncture steps	❑ Infectious disease interventions	❑ Shock therapeutic interventions	❑ Adjuvants	❑ Staging and grading	❑ Postoperative phase	❑ Frostbite
❑ Magnesium imbalances	❑ Nursing process	❑ Nursing process	❑ Nursing process	❑ WHO ladder	❑ Surgery	❑ Perianesthesia care unit	❑ Hyperthermia
❑ Acid–base balance	❑ Complications of IV therapy			❑ Routes for analgesic administration	❑ Radiation therapy	❑ Postoperative nursing care:	❑ Poisoning and drug overdose
❑ Respiratory acidosis	❑ Central venous access devices			❑ Nondrug therapies	❑ Chemo-therapy	❑ Respiratory	❑ Near-drowning
❑ Metabolic acidosis	❑ Nutrition support			❑ Nursing process	❑ Side effects of therapies	❑ Circulatory	❑ Psychiatric emergencies
❑ Respiratory alkalosis	❑ Home IV therapy			❑ Pain assessment	❑ Nursing process	❑ Pain	❑ Disaster response
❑ Metabolic alkalosis				❑ Patient education	❑ Hospice care	❑ Urinary	❑ Bioterrorism
					❑ Oncological emergencies	❑ Wound care	
						❑ Gastrointestinal	
						❑ Mobility	
						❑ Patient discharge	
						❑ Home health care	

6 Nursing Care of Patients With Fluid, Electrolyte, and Acid–Base Imbalances

VOCABULARY

Fill in the blanks with key terms from the chapter.

1. The process through which a solute moves from an area of higher to an area of lower concentration is
   _____.

2. A fluid that has the same osmolarity as blood is said to be _____.

3. A fluid that has a higher osmolarity than blood is said to be _____.

4. A decrease in blood volume is called _____.

5. Electrolytes in the blood that have a positive charge are called _____.

6. The patient with an excess of sodium in the blood has _____.

7. The patient with not enough potassium in the blood has _____.

8. The patient with not enough calcium in the blood has _____.

9. _____ occurs when the serum pH falls below 7.35.

10. If the serum pH is too high, the condition is called _____.

DEHYDRATION

Circle the errors in the following paragraph and write in the correct information.

Mrs. White is a 78-year-old woman admitted to the hospital with a diagnosis of severe dehydration. The licensed practical nurse/licensed vocational nurse (LPN/LVN) assigned to Mrs. White is asked to collect data related to fluid status. The LPN expects Mrs. White's blood pressure to be elevated because of the shift of fluid from tissues to her bloodstream. The nurse also finds Mrs. White's skin to be taut and firm and notes that the urine is copious and dark amber. The nurse asks Mrs. White if she knows where she is and what day it is because severe dehydration may cause confusion. In addition, the nurse initiates intake and output measurements because this is the most accurate way to monitor fluid balance.

ELECTROLYTE IMBALANCES

Match the electrolyte imbalance with its signs and symptoms.

1. _____ Hyponatremia
2. _____ Hyperkalemia
3. _____ Hypokalemia
4. _____ Hypercalcemia
5. _____ Hypocalcemia

1. Osteoporosis, hyperactive reflexes
2. Muscle weakness, weak pulse
3. Muscle weakness, kidney stones
4. Fluid balance and mental status changes
5. Muscle cramps, irregular heart rate

CRITICAL THINKING

Read the following case study and answer the questions.

Mr. James is an 89-year-old man admitted to your unit with worsening chronic bronchitis. On admission he is short of breath, but he is able to walk to the bathroom without difficulty. The physician orders bronchodilators, antibiotics, and an intravenous (IV) infusion of normal saline at 150 mL per hour. The next day when you return to work, you find Mr. James gasping for breath, coughing, and panicky. You quickly listen to his lungs and hear an increase in moist crackles since yesterday.

1. What additional data do you collect to confirm your suspicion of fluid overload?

   _____

   _____

   _____

   _____

2. You report your findings to the registered nurse (RN) and collaborate on quickly developing a nursing diagnosis of fluid overload. What factors contributed to this problem?

   _____

   _____

   _____

   _____

3. The RN pages the physician while you return to check on the patient. What nursing interventions can help until orders are received?

   _____

   _____

   _____

   _____

4. How will you know when the problem has been resolved?

   _____

   _____

   _____

REVIEW QUESTIONS—CONTENT REVIEW

Choose the best answer unless directed otherwise.

1. Which of the following IV solutions is hypotonic?
   1. Normal saline
   2. 0.45% saline
   3. Ringer's lactate
   4. 5% dextrose in normal saline

2. Which of the following hormones retains sodium in the body?
   1. Antidiuretic hormone
   2. Thyroid hormone
   3. Aldosterone
   4. Insulin

3. Which food should be avoided by the patient on a low-sodium diet?
   1. Apples
   2. Cheese
   3. Chicken
   4. Broccoli

4. Which food is recommended for the patient who must increase intake of potassium?
   1. Bread
   2. Egg
   3. Potato
   4. Cereal

5. Which is the most reliable method for monitoring fluid balance?
   1. Daily intake and output
   2. Daily weight
   3. Vital signs
   4. Skin turgor

6. An older adult patient presents to the emergency department reporting severe vomiting and diarrhea, sweating, and rapid heartbeat but has a normal temperature. In continuing the assessment of the patient, what should the nurse first suspect?
   1. Hypervolemia
   2. Dehydration
   3. Edema
   4. Hyponatremia

REVIEW QUESTIONS—TEST PREPARATION

Choose the best answer unless directed otherwise.

7. Which patient is most at risk for fluid volume overload?
   1. The 40-year-old with meningitis
   2. The 35-year-old with kidney failure
   3. The 60-year-old with psoriasis
   4. The 2-year-old with influenza

8. Which patients should be monitored closely for dehydration? **Select all that apply.**
   1. A 50-year-old with an ileostomy
   2. A 19-year-old with chronic asthma
   3. A 22-year-old with diabetes mellitus
   4. A 45-year-old with a temperature of 102.3°F
   5. A 28-year-old with a broken femur
   6. A 36-year-old taking diuretic therapy

9. An older-adult nursing home resident who has always been alert and oriented is now showing signs of dehydration and has become confused. Which electrolyte imbalance is most likely involved?
   1. Hyponatremia
   2. Hyperkalemia
   3. Hypercalcemia
   4. Hypomagnesemia

10. The LPN/LVN is caring for a patient with osteoporosis who appears weak and frail. Which of the following nursing interventions is best?
    1. Maintain bed rest
    2. Encourage fluids
    3. Ambulate with assistance
    4. Provide a high-protein diet

11. A 19-year-old student develops symptoms of respiratory alkalosis related to an anxiety attack. Which nursing intervention is most appropriate?
    1. Make sure his oxygen is being administered as ordered.
    2. Have him breathe into a paper bag.
    3. Place him in a semi-Fowler's position.
    4. Have him do coughing and deep-breathing exercises.

12. A patient has chronic respiratory acidosis related to long-standing lung disease. Which of the following problems is the cause?
    1. Hyperventilation
    2. Hypoventilation
    3. Loss of acid by kidneys
    4. Loss of base by kidneys

13. The nurse is providing discharge instructions for a patient taking Slow-K®, an oral potassium chloride supplement. Which of the following statements by the patient indicates that more teaching is needed? **Select all that apply.**
    1. "I won't use salt substitutes that have potassium."
    2. "I need to have my blood checked routinely."
    3. "I should take my supplement first thing in the morning and then wait 30 minutes before eating."
    4. "If the pill is too big to swallow, I can crush it."
    5. "I should call the doctor if I have nausea, vomiting, or abdominal cramps."
    6. "I can expect some diarrhea with this medication."

Nursing Care of Patients Receiving Intravenous Therapy

7

VOCABULARY

Match the term with the appropriate definition or statement.

1. _____ Intravenous (IV)
2. _____ Cannula
3. _____ Distal
4. _____ Infiltration
5. _____ Peripherally inserted central catheter (PICC)
6. _____ Hematoma
7. _____ Phlebitis
8. _____ Proximal

1. Inside a vein
2. Seepage of IV fluid into tissues
3. Nearest the point of attachment
4. Inflammation of a vein
5. Access device inserted into a superficial peripheral vein and advanced into the central system to the superior vena cava.
6. An IV needle or catheter with a stylet.
7. Farthest from the center or from the trunk
8. A localized collection of extravasated blood in the subcutaneous tissue, from a break in a blood vessel

PERIPHERAL VEINS

Label the veins that can be used for IV therapy.

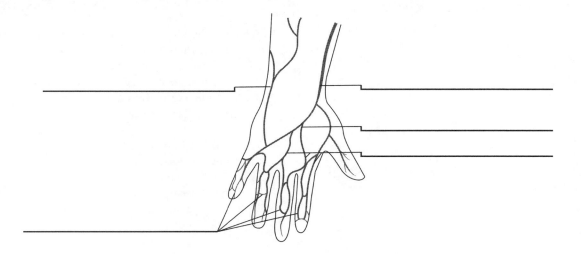

COMPLICATIONS OF IV THERAPY

Fill in the blank with the correct complication.

1. Pain and inflammation at the IV insertion site is called _____.

2. Redness and exudate at the IV insertion site indicate the presence of _____.

3. Infiltration into tissue by an IV fluid or drug is called _____.

4. Dyspnea and crackles can be a sign of _____ _____.

5. A cool, puffy insertion site indicates _____.

6. Fever, chills, and tachycardia indicate a systemic infection called _____.

7. Sharp pain at the IV site during infusion of a cold fluid indicates a _____.

8. If the patient develops cyanosis, hypotension, and loss of consciousness, the nurse should suspect _____ _____.

CRITICAL THINKING

Read the following case study and answer the questions.

Mr. Livesay is admitted with cellulitis and is receiving IV fluids by gravity drip. When you check his IV, you find it is not dripping. What data can you collect to determine the cause of the problem? What is the role of the licensed practical nurse (LPN)? When must the registered nurse (RN) be consulted? _____ _____ _____ _____ _____

CALCULATION PRACTICE

Calculate the answers to the following problems. Round each answer to the nearest whole number.

1. June has an IV of 5% dextrose in water ordered to infuse at 83 mL/hr. How many drops per minute should be set if the tubing delivers 15 drops per milliliter?

2. Frank has a piggyback antibiotic of 500 mg in 50 mL of 5% dextrose in water. The medication must infuse over 20 minutes. The tubing drip factor is 10. How many drops per minute?

3. Dave has an IV of normal saline ordered at 1 L over 12 hours. How many milliliters per hour should he receive?

4. Lucy has an order to administer 800 units of heparin per hour. The registered nurse hangs heparin 50,000 units in 500 mL of 5% dextrose in water. It will run on an electronic infusion device. How many milliliters should be administered per hour?

5. Jack has an order for 1000 mL of normal saline over 24 hours. How many drops should be administered per minute, using microdrop tubing?

REVIEW QUESTIONS—CONTENT REVIEW

Choose the best answer unless directed otherwise.

1. Which vein should be used first when initiating IV therapy?
   1. Jugular
   2. Basilic
   3. Brachiocephalic
   4. Axillary

2. When preparing a site for venipuncture with chlorhexidine gluconate, how long must the area be cleaned?
   1. 5 seconds
   2. 10 seconds
   3. 30 seconds
   4. 60 seconds

3. Which of the following complications can occur if a clotted cannula is aggressively flushed?
   1. A clot can enter the circulation.
   2. An air embolism can enter the circulation.
   3. A painful arterial spasm can occur.
   4. The patient can experience speed shock.

4. Which of the following symptoms most likely indicates that an infusion is infiltrated?
   1. Redness at the site
   2. Pain at the site
   3. Puffiness at the site
   4. Exudate at the site

5. An 87-year-old patient recovering from abdominal surgery has a continuous IV infusion to supply nutrients and antibiotics. What complication should the LPN suspect when signs and symptoms of redness, warmth, and pain at the infusion site are reported?
   1. Phlebitis
   2. Thrombosis
   3. Hematoma
   4. Infiltration

REVIEW QUESTIONS—TEST PREPARATION

Choose the best answer unless directed otherwise.

6. Which patient would benefit most from a capped IV access that is used intermittently rather than continuously?
   1. The patient with pneumonia who needs fluids and antibiotics
   2. The patient who has had major blood loss after a motor vehicle accident
   3. The young child who is dehydrated
   4. The older patient who is receiving a diuretic for fluid overload

7. The physician orders furosemide (Lasix) 40 mg IV push (IVP) STAT for a patient in acute fluid overload. Why was the IV route likely chosen?
   1. Furosemide can be administered only by the IV route.
   2. IVP is the route of choice for rapid action.
   3. IVP dosing is more accurate.
   4. IVP furosemide has fewer side effects than oral.

8. A patient has orders to receive 1 L (1000 mL) of 5% dextrose and lactated Ringer's solution to be infused over 8 hours. How many milliliters will be infused per hour?
   1. 80
   2. 100
   3. 125
   4. 150

9. A patient is receiving an IV piggyback antibiotic in 50 mL of 5% dextrose in water to run over 1 hour. The tubing has a drop factor of 60. How many drops per minute should be delivered?
   1. 6
   2. 17
   3. 50
   4. 100

10. The nurse is caring for a patient who is to receive IV fluids at 100 mL per hour with IV antibiotic therapy scheduled every 4 hours. Which of the following sites for the IV placement is best?
    1. Large vein on the dorsal side of the patient's nondominant arm
    2. Small vein on the surface of the patient's dominant hand
    3. Small vein on the surface of the patient's nondominant hand
    4. Large vein in the nondominant antecubital space

8

Nursing Care of Patients With Infections

VOCABULARY

Define the following terms and use them in a sentence.

Antigen

Definition: _____

Sentence: _____

Asepsis

Definition: _____

Sentence: _____

Bacteria

Definition: _____

Sentence: _____

Clostridium difficile (C. diff)

Definition: _____

Sentence: _____

Hand hygiene

Definition: _____

Sentence: _____

Pathogens

Definition: _____

Sentence: _____

Personal protective equipment

Definition: _____

Sentence: _____

Phagocytosis

Definition: _____

Sentence: _____

Sepsis

Definition: _____

Sentence: _____

Virulence

Definition: _____

Sentence: _____

Viruses

Definition: _____

Sentence: _____

PATHOGEN TRANSMISSION

Match the pathogen with its mode of transmission.

1. _____ Chickenpox
2. _____ Malaria
3. _____ Tuberculosis
4. _____ Rocky Mountain spotted fever
5. _____ Meningitis
6. _____ Pneumonia
7. _____ Measles
8. _____ Influenza
9. _____ Pneumonic plague
10. _____ Hepatitis A

1. Common vehicle
2. Droplet
3. Airborne
4. Vectorborne

PATHOGENS AND INFECTIOUS DISEASE

Fill in the blanks with the appropriate pathogen or infectious disease name.

1. _____ Gram-positive bacteria clusters that can cause pneumonia, cellulitis, peritonitis, and toxic shock.

2. _____ Group of plantlike organisms that includes yeast, molds, and mushrooms; rarely pathogenic.

3. _____ A fungi that can cause thrush.

4. _____ The virus that causes infectious mononucleosis.

5. _____ A systemic fungal respiratory disease caused by *Histoplasma capsulatum*.

6. _____ A disease caused by infection with the protozoan *Toxoplasma gondii*.

7. _____ Single-celled parasitic organisms that move and live mainly in the soil.

8. _____ Small intracellular parasites that can only live inside cells; may produce disease when they enter a cell.

9. _____ A bacterium that must be inside living cells to reproduce and cause disease and causes Rocky Mountain spotted fever.

10. _____ Bleach is used to kill its spores.

CRITICAL THINKING

Read the following case study and answer the questions.

A 72-year-old patient is admitted to a private room with an antibiotic-resistant respiratory tract infection.

1. What equipment is needed for isolation? _____

_____

_____

_____

2. What type of equipment would be used to do assessments and nursing interventions?

_____

_____

_____

3. Describe the psychosocial effects on a patient in isolation.

_____

_____

_____

4. What can the nurse include in the plan of care for a patient in isolation to reduce social isolation?

_____

_____

_____

5. What condition is the patient at risk of developing during antibiotic treatment for this infection?

_____

_____

_____

6. What intervention can be used to reduce this risk during antibiotic treatment?

_____

_____

_____

REVIEW QUESTIONS—CONTENT REVIEW

Choose the best answer unless directed otherwise.

1. Which of the following would the nurse recognize as a sign of a local infection during data collection?
   1. Warm skin
   2. Clammy skin
   3. Anorexia
   4. Paleness

2. Which of the following does the nurse understand is a sterile technique method?
   1. Use of antiseptics
   2. Use of autoclaves
   3. Frequent hand washing
   4. Use of gloves when coming in contact with body fluids

3. Which of the following infections would the nurse recognize as being a health care–acquired infection?
   1. Chronic urinary tract infection for a homebound person
   2. A sexually transmitted infection in a healthy young adult
   3. Pneumonia in a hospitalized postoperative patient
   4. Hospitalization for cellulitis

4. Which of the following antibiotics would the nurse anticipate would be used to treat methicillin-resistant *Staphylococcus aureus* (MRSA)?
   1. Gentamicin
   2. Tobramycin
   3. Penicillin
   4. Vancomycin

5. A nurse should wear a fit-tested high-efficiency particulate air filter (HEPA) mask when entering the room of a patient with which disease?
   1. Influenza
   2. Scabies
   3. HIV infection
   4. Tuberculosis

REVIEW QUESTIONS—TEST PREPARATION

Choose the best answer unless directed otherwise.

6. Which of the following actions would be MOST appropriate for the nurse to take while providing patient care to help prevent the spread of infection?
   1. Sterilizing hands with a germicide once a day
   2. Washing hands at the beginning of patient rounds
   3. Performing hand hygiene before and after each patient contact
   4. Wearing gloves for all patient care

7. In planning care for a patient, the nurse understands that surgical asepsis is based on which of the following principles?
   1. Destroying organisms before they enter the body
   2. Isolating all patients who have infectious diseases
   3. Destroying bacteria as they leave the body
   4. Maintaining basic cleanliness

8. Which of the following does the nurse understand is needed by all pathogenic organisms to multiply? **Select all that apply.**
   1. Moisture
   2. Light
   3. A host
   4. Oxygen
   5. Warmth
   6. Food

9. A patient is to have a sterile urine specimen collected. Which of the following techniques is used to collect this specimen? **Select all that apply.**
   1. Cleansing the patient's external genitalia before the patient voids
   2. Having the patient void into a sterile container
   3. Straight catheterizing the patient
   4. Obtaining a midstream voided specimen
   5. Obtaining a second voiding specimen
   6. Placing urine specimen from catheter in a sterile container

10. Which of the following actions can the nurse take to help prevent a health care–acquired infection in an incontinent patient?
    1. Avoiding use of a urinary catheter
    2. Applying absorbent briefs
    3. Toileting patient every 4 hours
    4. Restricting fluids

11. A patient has been diagnosed recently as having an upper respiratory infection. Which of the following symptoms would indicate to the nurse that the patient is developing a complication?
    1. Scratchy throat
    2. Clear, watery drainage from the nose
    3. Dry cough
    4. High fever

12. The nurse is collecting a culture of wound drainage, and the patient asks what a culture is. Which of the following is the best response by the nurse to explain what a culture is?
    1. A culture identifies the presence of pathogens.
    2. A culture measures antibiotic levels.
    3. A culture identifies an antibiotic's effect on a pathogen.
    4. A culture determines the appropriate medication dosage.

13. Which of the following data collection findings should the nurse recognize and report as a possible sign of infection in the older adult? **Select all that apply.**
    1. Poor skin turgor
    2. Irritability
    3. Hypertension
    4. Bradycardia
    5. Pacing behavior
    6. Hunger

14. The nurse observes a nursing assistant providing oral care to an immunocompromised patient. The use of which of the following by the nursing assistant would require further instruction for patient safety?
    1. Sterile water
    2. Tap water
    3. Fluoride toothpaste
    4. Soft toothbrush

9

Nursing Care of Patients in Shock

VOCABULARY

Fill in the blank with the word formed by word building.

1. _____ acid—sour + osis—condition
2. _____ an—without + aerobic—presence of oxygen
3. _____ an—without + phylaxis—protection
4. _____ dys—difficult + rhythmia—rhythm
5. _____ kardia—heart + genesis—beginning
6. _____ cyan—blue coloring + osis—condition
7. _____ tachy—fast + pnea—breathing
8. _____ olig—few + uria—urine condition
9. _____ tachy—fast + cardia—heart condition
10. _____ hypo-low + perfuser—to pour over or through

MATCHING

Match the area of the cardiovascular system that contributes to the development of shock with each type of shock.

1. _____ Hypovolemic shock
2. _____ Cardiogenic shock
3. _____ Anaphylactic shock
4. _____ Septic shock
5. _____ Neurogenic shock
6. _____ Obstructive shock

1. Heart
2. Blood vessels
3. Fluid volume

SIGNS AND SYMPTOMS OF SHOCK PHASES

Complete the table.

Signs/Symptoms	Phases		
	Compensating	**Progressive**	**Irreversible**
Heart rate	Elevated		Slowing
Pulses	_____	Weaker, thready	_____
Systolic Blood pressure	Normal	<90 mm Hg	_____
		*In hypertensive, 25% below baseline	
Diastolic Blood pressure	_____	_____	Decreasing to 0
Respirations	_____	Tachypnea	_____
Depth	_____		_____
Temperature	Varies	Decreased	_____
		*May elevate in septic shock	
Level of consciousness	_____	Confused, lethargy	Unconscious, comatose
Skin/mucous membranes	Cool, pale	Cold, moist, clammy, pale	_____
Urine output	_____	_____	15 mL/hr decreasing to anuria
Bowel sounds	_____	Decreasing	_____

CRITICAL THINKING

Identify the stage of shock, category of shock, and initial action to take for the following patients.

1. An 80-year-old woman admitted with a bowel obstruction has minimal urine output. A nasogastric tube has 1500 mL of bloody aspirate returned on insertion. She becomes comatose. Vital signs are as follows: blood pressure 78 mm Hg with Doppler stethoscope, pulse 140 beats per minute and thready, respirations 8 per minute, and temperature 94°F (34°C).
   Stage: _____
   Category of Shock: _____
   Initial Action: _____

2. A 56-year-old patient with chronic renal failure is agitated. Her blood pressure is 100/92 mm Hg, pulse 110 beats per minute, respirations 18 per minute, and temperature 102°°F (39°C).
   Stage: _____
   Category of Shock: _____
   Initial Action: _____

3. A 50-year-old patient who is hypotensive is receiving a fluid challenge of 1000 mL 0.9% normal saline over 4 hours. Her lung sounds are now full of crackles. Her heart rhythm is irregular. Jugular vein distention and ankle edema are present. Blood pressure has dropped from 96/50 to 80/40 mm Hg in 1 hour, pulse 108 beats per minute, respirations 24 per minute, and temperature 95°F (35°C). She is confused.
   Stage: _____
   Category of Shock: _____
   Initial Action: _____

REVIEW QUESTIONS—CONTENT REVIEW

Choose the best answer unless directed otherwise.

1. Which of the following nursing interventions would the nurse use to collect data to determine status of peripheral tissue perfusion in a 48-year-old patient in shock?
   1. Obtain apical pulse.
   2. Check capillary refill.
   3. Check for sacral edema.
   4. Monitor level of consciousness.

2. Which of the following does the nurse understand is the primary reason that respirations increase in compensated shock?
   1. Anxiety causes hyperventilation.
   2. Retention of carbon dioxide is decreased.
   3. Normal oxygen levels are maintained.
   4. Cardiac output is increased.

3. With which of the following types of shock would the nurse anticipate the skin to be cold and moist during data collection?
   1. Compensating
   2. Progressive
   3. Irreversible

4. The nurse is caring for a hypertensive patient whose blood pressure is usually 156/86. Which of the following blood pressures is considered a progressive shock blood pressure finding for this patient?
   1. 90/44
   2. 140/80
   3. 114/64
   4. 130/72

5. Which of the following outcomes for the nursing diagnosis *Deficient Knowledge* is appropriate for the patient recovering from shock?
   1. Accepts responsibility for shock
   2. States understanding of shock
   3. Interacts with others
   4. Verbalizes fears

REVIEW QUESTIONS—TEST PREPARATION

Choose the best answer unless directed otherwise.

6. The nurse monitors a patient with chronic kidney disease who has just returned from completing a hemodialysis session. The patient's data before dialysis is as follows: blood pressure 150/88 mm Hg, pulse 90 beats per minute, respirations 18 per minute, temperature 98.9°F (37°C), and weight 168 lb. Patient data obtained after dialysis is as follows: blood pressure 98/50 mm Hg, pulse 110 beats per minute, respirations 18 per minute, temperature 99°F (37°C), and weight 165 lb. Which of the following actions should the nurse take after comparing the data?
   1. Reweigh the patient.
   2. Provide a quiet environment so patient may rest.
   3. Have the health care provider notified of the post-dialysis data.
   4. Check on the patient in 10 minutes.

7. A 47-year-old patient is admitted with hypovolemic shock from trauma injuries resulting from an automobile accident. The patient remains oliguric 2 days later. Which of the following assessments of the patient indicates to the nurse that the patient is experiencing a complication of shock that requires follow-up treatment?
   1. Hematocrit 42% (normal = 38%–47%)
   2. Creatinine 2.2 mg/dL (normal = 0.6–1.3 mg/dL)
   3. Blood urea nitrogen 24 mg/dL (normal = 6–25 mg/dL)
   4. Hemoglobin 13.4 g/dL (normal = 13.5–18 g/dL)

8. The nurse is caring for a patient with a bowel obstruction. Which of the following is the earliest indication that the patient is developing symptoms of shock?
   1. Blood pressure 88/50 mm Hg
   2. Pulse 110 beats per minute
   3. Lethargy
   4. Urine 18 mL/hr

9. The nurse is caring for a postoperative patient following a splenectomy. Which of the following symptoms is of highest priority for the nurse to report?
   1. Blood pressure 86/52 mm Hg
   2. Pulse 100 beats per minute
   3. Cool, pale skin
   4. Urine 40 mL/hr

10. The nurse is caring for a patient with gastrointestinal bleeding who has an intravenous (IV) infusion of 0.9% normal saline at 50 mL/hr. The patient has a large, red, bloody stool and reports dizziness. The nurse assists the patient back to bed and obtains vital signs of blood pressure 90/52 mm Hg, pulse 118 beats per minute, and respirations 22 per minute. Which of the following actions should the nurse take?
    1. Continue monitoring vital signs.
    2. Inform the registered nurse now.
    3. Decrease the IV flow rate.
    4. Elevate the head of the bed.

11. Which of the following medications would the nurse anticipate the health care provider may order to increase blood pressure for a patient with septic shock?
    1. Atropine
    2. Dopamine
    3. Digoxin (Lanoxin)
    4. Nitroglycerin

12. For the patient in hypovolemic shock, place the following interventions in the order of priority in which the nurse should perform them.
    1. Record hourly urine output.
    2. Apply oxygen.
    3. Provide restful environment.
    4. Ensure patent airway.
    5. Obtain vital signs.
    6. Monitor IV fluids.

13. The nurse is providing care for a patient with pericardial effusion who is at risk for pericardial tamponade. Which of the following symptoms would indicate the patient was developing obstructive shock? **Select all that apply.**
    1. BP 88/56 mm Hg
    2. Urine output 100 mL over 6 hours
    3. Pulse 66 beats per minute
    4. Respirations 12 per minute
    5. Jugular vein distension
    6. Confusion and lethargy

Nursing Care of Patients in Pain

VOCABULARY

Match the term with the appropriate definition or statement.

1. _____ Addiction
2. _____ Tolerance
3. _____ Ceiling effect
4. _____ Pain
5. _____ Prostaglandin
6. _____ Adjuvants
7. _____ Opioid
8. _____ Patient-controlled anesthesia (PCA)
9. _____ Endorphins
10. _____ Analgesics

1. Whatever the experiencing person says it is
2. Endogenous chemicals that act like opioids
3. Larger dose of analgesic required to relieve same pain
4. Psychological dependence
5. Self-administered analgesics
6. Dose of analgesic limited by side effects
7. Medications that relieve pain
8. Drugs that are used to potentiate analgesics
9. Neurotransmitter released during pain
10. A morphine-like drug

CULTURAL COMPETENCE

You are working on a medical unit in a large metropolitan area. Your patients come from varied cultural backgrounds. What differences in pain expressions might you expect to see in patients from the following cultures?

Native American _____

European American _____

African American _____

Hispanic American _____

Asian American _____

Arab American _____

CRITICAL THINKING

Read the following case study and answer the questions.

Ms. Murphy is a 32-year-old woman admitted to your unit following an emergency appendectomy at 0800. When you enter her room at 1400, she is sitting up in bed smiling and visiting with her family. She tells you she is hurting and asks for her pain medication. You check her medication record and find orders for morphine 5 to 10 mg intravenous push (IVP) every 4 hours as needed (prn) for pain.

1. List at least seven areas you will assess related to her pain. _____

   _____

   _____

   _____

2. Based on your assessment, you discuss administering 10 mg of morphine with the registered nurse (RN), who will give the intravenous (IV) medication. What class of drugs does morphine belong to? What is its mechanism of action? Why is it important for you to be aware of these things when the RN is administering the drug?

   _____

   _____

   _____

   _____

3. What is the most effective medication schedule that can be implemented today? _____

_____

_____

4. What side effects will you watch for? _____

_____

_____

5. How will you know if the medication has been effective?

_____

_____

_____

_____

6. The next morning you decide to administer Tylenol #3 (acetaminophen 300 mg with codeine 30 mg) for Ms. Murphy's pain, but it is not effective. Why do you think it did not help? _____

_____

_____

7. What nondrug therapies might be appropriate for Ms. Murphy? What technique has already been effective for her? _____

_____

_____

_____

REVIEW QUESTIONS—CONTENT REVIEW

Choose the best answer unless directed otherwise.

1. Which of the following definitions of pain is most appropriate to use when planning nursing care?
   1. Knifelike sensation along a nerve pathway
   2. Burning sensation that accompanies severe injury or trauma
   3. Injured tissues responding with release of neurotransmitters that cause a sensation of pressure or discomfort
   4. Whatever the experiencing person says it is, occurring whenever the person experiencing it says it does

2. Which of the following terms describes a feeling of threat to one's self-image or life that may accompany pain?
   1. Fear
   2. Anxiety
   3. Suffering
   4. Panic

3. Which of the following is a common side effect of opioid administration?
   1. Constipation
   2. Respiratory depression
   3. Tachycardia
   4. Addiction

4. Which is the most accurate way to assess the severity of a patient's pain?
   1. Observe for moaning or other physical signs.
   2. Watch for elevated blood pressure and pulse.
   3. Have the patient rate pain on a standard pain scale.
   4. Monitor the frequency with which the patient requests pain medication.

5. Which of the following statements best explains why a patient can be laughing and talking and yet still be in pain?
   1. Most patients try to deny their pain because pain is socially unacceptable.
   2. Distraction can help relieve pain when used in combination with analgesics.
   3. Most patients who are laughing and talking are not in pain.
   4. Laughing prolongs the effects of opioids in the body.

REVIEW QUESTIONS—TEST PREPARATION

Choose the best answer unless directed otherwise.

6. An 82-year-old patient in an extended care facility has been receiving intramuscular (IM) meperidine (Demerol) for chronic back pain. After several weeks, the patient becomes irritable, which is a change from normal behavior. Which response by the nurse is best?
   1. Understand that chronic pain can cause a patient to become irritable.
   2. Obtain an order for an adjuvant sedative to administer with the meperidine.
   3. Request a psychiatric referral to evaluate the patient's mental status.
   4. Consult with the RN or health care provider about changing to a different analgesic.

7. A nurse is caring for a patient who reports being in severe pain. The patient has an order for hydrocodone/acetaminophen (Vicodin) 2 tabs every 6 hours prn for pain. Before providing the medication, which of the following actions should the nurse take?
   1. Verify the patient's liver and kidney function studies are within normal limits.
   2. Determine the patient's current pulse rate and blood glucose level.
   3. Assess the patient's pain level and respiratory rate.
   4. Identify the emotional or physical cause of the patient's pain.

8. A patient with severe pain is receiving narcotic pain medication through the use of a patient-controlled analgesia IV pump. The licensed practical nurse/licensed vocational nurse (LPN/LVN) notes that the patient is lethargic and difficult to arouse with a respiratory rate of seven breaths per minute. After informing the RN, which of the following drugs does the nurse anticipate will be ordered?
   1. Naloxone (Narcan)
   2. Methadone (Dolophine)
   3. Hydrocodone with acetaminophen (Vicodin)
   4. Phenytoin (Dilantin)

9. A 42-year-old woman has chronic pain for which no cause can be found. Her physician orders a placebo. Which response by the nurse to the physician is best?
   1. "I will give the placebo and document her response."
   2. "I know if the placebo helps her pain, then her pain is not real."
   3. "I am not comfortable administering this placebo without the patient's consent."
   4. "May we alternate the placebo with her opioid order?"

10. A patient has a PCA pump after surgery on his spine. He appears to be in pain but is too drowsy to push the button on the pump. Which response by the nurse is correct?
    1. Push the button for the patient.
    2. Instruct the patient's wife to push the button, not to exceed every 10 minutes.
    3. Assess the patient's vital signs.
    4. Increase the dose of medication delivered in each injection.

11. A patient with a known history of cocaine abuse is admitted after a motorcycle accident. He calls you into his room and says, "I need something for this pain. Now." Which assumption by the nurse is best?
    1. The patient is withdrawing from cocaine and needs an opioid to prevent withdrawal symptoms.
    2. The patient is in pain and needs an analgesic.
    3. The patient is trying to establish control over his situation.
    4. The patient is faking pain to gain access to opioids.

12. The nurse is providing care for a patient in the emergency department who is experiencing a migraine headache. The patient reports taking two extra-strength acetaminophen (Tylenol 500 mg tablets) every 6 hours for the past few days. The nurse would be most concerned by which of the following statements by the patient?
    1. "I usually drink three or four beers a day."
    2. "My headache pain is six out of ten."
    3. "I'm having difficulty sleeping."
    4. "It hurts even worse with these bright lights."

Nursing Care of Patients With Cancer

11

VOCABULARY

Fill in the blank.

1. Loss of hair is called _____.
2. Loss of appetite is called _____.
3. _____ places the patient at risk of infection.
4. Dry mouth is called _____.
5. Treatment aimed at maintaining comfort is called _____ therapy.
6. _____ is the use of drugs to combat cancer.
7. Substances that poison cells are described as _____.
8. _____ is the term used to describe new growth.
9. When cancer _____, it travels to a new site.
10. A tumor that is not cancerous is called _____.
11. A _____ is done to obtain a tissue sample to detect cancer cells.
12. Agents that prevent damage to healthy cells from chemotherapy or radiation are called _____ agents.

CELLS

Label each statement as true or false and correct the false statement.

1. _____ Chromosomes are made of DNA and protein.
2. _____ A gene is the code for one DNA molecule.
3. _____ Messenger RNA carries the genetic code to the cell membrane.
4. _____ A genetic change in a cell is called a mutation.
5. _____ Transfer RNA brings amino acids to the proper sites on the DNA.
6. _____ Cells become malignant by mutating.
7. _____ In any human cell, most of the genes are always active.
8. _____ The chromosome number for a human cell is 48.
9. _____ The process of mitosis produces two identical cells with 23 chromosomes each.
10. _____ Mitosis is necessary only for growth of the body.

BENIGN VERSUS MALIGNANT TUMORS

Compare the characteristics of benign and malignant tumors. List as many characteristics as you can remember.

_____

_____

_____

_____

_____

CRITICAL THINKING

Delmae is a 48-year-old restaurant worker undergoing chemotherapy following a right modified mastectomy. List two or three nursing interventions for each of the side effects she can expect to experience.

1. Leukopenia: _____

_____

2. Thrombocytopenia: _____

_____

3. Anemia: _____

_____

4. Stomatitis: _____

_____

5. Nausea and vomiting: _____

_____

6. Alopecia: _____

_____

REVIEW QUESTIONS—CONTENT REVIEW

Choose the best answer unless directed otherwise.

1. Genes are made of which of the following?
   1. Chromosomes
   2. DNA
   3. RNA
   4. Protein

2. Which is the correct term used for a group of similar cells found on an external or internal body surface?
   1. Skin
   2. Mucous membrane
   3. Epithelial tissue
   4. Connective tissue

3. Which of the following foods can increase cancer risk?
   1. Broccoli, cauliflower
   2. Butter, ice cream
   3. Chicken, fish
   4. Cakes, breads

4. A nurse is caring for a patient with a radioactive implant. How can the nurse avoid unnecessary radiation exposure?
   1. Avoid entering the patient's room more than once each 24 hours.
   2. Limit the amount of time spent with the patient.
   3. Avoid touching the patient.
   4. Place a "contaminated" sign on the patient's bed.

Choose the best answer unless directed otherwise.

5. A patient is admitted with suspected lung cancer and asks, "How will my physician know for sure if I have cancer?" Which of the following responses is correct?
   1. "Your physician will do cultures of your sputum."
   2. "An X-ray examination will be done to confirm the diagnosis."
   3. "A biopsy is the only way to know for sure."
   4. "Your physician will do a bronchoscopy to view the cancer."

6. Which of the following nursing interventions will help relieve symptoms of mucositis related to radiation therapy?
   1. Provide frequent mouth care.
   2. Offer cold liquids often.
   3. Provide high-carbohydrate foods.
   4. Offer juices frequently.

7. A patient is receiving chemotherapy after surgery for prostate cancer. Which of the following signs or symptoms indicates that he is experiencing thrombocytopenia?
   1. Fever
   2. Petechiae
   3. Pain
   4. Vomiting

8. How can the nurse best prevent complications in the patient with leukopenia? **Select all that apply.**
   1. Wash hands frequently.
   2. Avoid injections.
   3. Allow no visitors.
   4. Provide colony stimulating factors as ordered.
   5. Monitor temperature every 4 hours.
   6. Offer fresh fruits and vegetables.

9. A patient has severe pain related to bone cancer. The nurse notes that the patient does not ask for pain medication while watching television. Which of the following statements best explains this?
   1. Distraction is a good pain relief method and can prevent the need for analgesics.
   2. The patient may ask for pain medication when the television is not on because of boredom.
   3. The pain must be psychosomatic because it is relieved by television.
   4. Distraction can be a helpful intervention when used in addition to analgesics.

10. A patient with terminal cancer is referred to hospice for support. How can hospice help the patient and family? **Select all that apply.**
    1. Hospice nurses can help administer curative chemotherapy.
    2. Hospice supports research efforts in finding cancer cures.
    3. Hospice can help the patient's family keep the patient comfortable until death.
    4. Hospice can help the patient find financial resources for cancer treatment.
    5. Hospice can provide follow-up counseling after the patient's death.
    6. Hospice can provide respite care for family members or caregivers.

11. The nurse is providing care for a patient in an outpatient surgical center anticipating a needle biopsy of suspicious nodules in the left lung. The patient asks, "If they think this might be cancer, why don't they just cut it all out?" Which of the following responses by the nurse is best?
    1. "Most patients who have lung biopsies don't end up having cancer."
    2. "Why do they think you have cancer?"
    3. "The biopsy will determine if you have cancer and, if so, what treatment is best."
    4. "It does seem odd that the doctor didn't simply schedule surgery."

12

Nursing Care of Patients Having Surgery

VOCABULARY

Fill in the blank.

1. _____ are physicians who perform surgical procedures.

2. The three surgical phases are referred to collectively by the term _____.

3. The _____ phase begins with the admission of the patient to the perianesthesia care unit (PACU) and continues until the patient's recovery is completed.

4. _____ is the period when an anesthetic is first given until full anesthesia is reached.

5. The _____ phase begins with the decision to have surgery and ends with transfer of the patient to the operating room.

6. The _____ phase begins when the patient is transferred to the operating room and ends when the patient is admitted to the PACU.

7. An _____ agent is medication (such as narcotics, muscle relaxants, or antiemetics) used with the primary anesthetic agents.

8. The sudden bursting open of a wound's edges that may be preceded by an increase in serosanguineous drainage is referred to as _____.

9. _____ are physicians who administer anesthesia.

10. _____ causes a loss of sensation and allows the surgical procedure to be done safely.

11. _____ occurs from hypoventilation or mucous obstruction that prevents some alveoli from opening and being fully ventilated.

12. _____ is the removal of necrotic and infected tissue.

13. _____ is a body temperature that is below normal range.

14. _____ is the viscera spilling out of the abdomen.

SURGERY URGENCY LEVELS

Match the surgery urgency level to the appropriate definition or example. The level may be used more than once.

1. _____ Surgery needed when any delay jeopardizes the patient's life or limb
2. _____ Fracture repair
3. _____ Surgery needed within 24 to 30 hours
4. _____ Extremity emboli
5. _____ Surgery planned and scheduled without immediate time constraints
6. _____ Surgery done at request of patient
7. _____ Hernia repair
8. _____ Rhinoplasty
9. _____ Infected gallbladder
10. _____ Cosmetic surgery

1. Optional surgery
2. Elective surgery
3. Urgent surgery
4. Emergency surgery

NOURISHING THE SURGICAL PATIENT

Find the seven errors and insert the correct information.

Healing requires increased vitamin A for collagen formation, vitamin B_{12} for blood clotting, and magnesium for tissue growth, skin integrity, and cell-mediated immunity. Carbohydrates are essential for controlling fluid balance and manufacturing antibodies and white blood cells. Hypoalbuminemia, low urine albumin, impedes the return of interstitial fluid to the venous return system, decreasing the risk of shock. A serum zinc level is a useful measure of protein status.

MEDICATIONS

Indicate whether the statement is true or false and correct the false statement.

1. _____ All medications that patients are taking must be reviewed preoperatively.
2. _____ Most anticoagulants, such as warfarin (Coumadin), do not need to be stopped before surgery.
3. _____ Diabetic patients on insulin are told to increase their normal insulin dose the day of surgery.
4. _____ Blood glucose monitoring for diabetic patients is ordered on admission.
5. _____ If a patient is on chronic oral steroid therapy, it cannot be abruptly stopped when nil per os (NPO).
6. _____ Surgery is not a serious stressor for the body.
7. _____ Chronic oral steroid therapy should be continued via the parenteral route if the patient is NPO.
8. _____ Circulatory collapse can develop if steroids are not stopped abruptly.

INTRAOPERATIVE NURSING DIAGNOSES AND OUTCOMES

Write a patient objective (goal) for each nursing diagnosis.

1. *Risk for Injury* related to pressure points from positioning, chemicals, electrical equipment, and effect of being anesthetized _____

   _____

2. *Risk for Impaired Skin Integrity* related to chemicals, pressure points from positioning, and immobility

   _____

   _____

3. *Risk for Deficient Fluid Volume* related to being NPO and blood loss _____

   _____

4. *Risk for Infection* related to incision and invasive procedures _____

   _____

5. *Pain* related to pressure points from positioning, incision, and surgical procedure _____

   _____

   _____

WOUND HEALING PHASES

Complete the table.

Phase	Time Frame	Wound Healing	Patient Effect
Phase I	_____		Fever, malaise
Phase II	_____	Granulation tissue forms	_____
Phase III	_____	Collagen deposited	_____
Phase IV	Months to 1 year	_____	_____

CRITICAL THINKING

Read the case study and answer the questions.

Mrs. Vell, 74, is scheduled for a total hip replacement because of osteoarthritis. She is seen in the preadmission testing department 1 week before surgery.

1. Why is Mrs. Vell being seen in preadmission testing?

   _____

   _____

   _____

2. What preadmission testing may be done?

   _____

   _____

   _____

3. What teaching should the nurse do in preadmission testing?

   _____

   _____

   _____

4. What are the responsibilities of the admitting nurse to prepare Mrs. Vell for surgery?

   _____

   _____

   _____

5. What is the role of the holding area nurse?

   _____

   _____

   _____

6. What is a role of the licensed practical nurse/licensed vocational nurse (LPN/LVN) in the operating room?

   _____

   _____

   _____

7. What are the two prioritized primary responsibilities of the perianesthesia care nurse?

   _____

   _____

   _____

8. Explain why postoperative care for this patient includes pain control, deep breathing and coughing, leg exercises, activity, leg abduction, and drain care.

   _____

   _____

   _____

   _____

   _____

   _____

   _____

REVIEW QUESTIONS—CONTENT REVIEW

Choose the best answer unless directed otherwise.

1. Which of the following is an LPN/LVN patient care role in the preoperative phase?
   1. Obtaining preoperative orders
   2. Explaining the surgical procedure
   3. Offering emotional support
   4. Providing informed consent

2. When the patient's signature is witnessed by the nurse on the surgical consent, which of the following does the nurse's signature indicate?
   1. The nurse obtained informed consent.
   2. The nurse provided informed consent.
   3. The nurse answered all surgical procedure questions.
   4. The nurse verified that the patient signed the consent.

3. Which of the following is an intraoperative outcome for a patient undergoing an inguinal hernia repair?
   1. Verbalizes fears.
   2. Maintains skin integrity.
   3. Demonstrates leg exercises.
   4. Explains deep-breathing exercises.

4. Which of the following is a discharge criterion from the PACU for a patient after surgery?
   1. Oxygen saturation above 90%
   2. Oxygen saturation below 90%
   3. Intravenous (IV) narcotics given less than 15 minutes earlier
   4. IV narcotics given less than 30 minutes earlier

5. Which of the following is one of the discharge criteria from ambulatory surgery for patients following surgery?
   1. Able to drive self home.
   2. Has home telephone.
   3. Understands discharge instructions.
   4. IV narcotics given less than 30 minutes before discharge.

REVIEW QUESTIONS—TEST PREPARATION

Choose the best answer unless directed otherwise.

6. The LPN/LVN is caring for a patient in the preoperative period who, even after verbalizing concerns and having questions answered, states, "I know I am not going to wake up after surgery." Which of the following actions should the LPN/LVN take?
   1. Reassure patient everything will be all right.
   2. Inform the registered nurse.
   3. Explain national surgery death rate.
   4. Ask family to comfort the patient.

7. The nurse understands that which of the following is the reason that long-term steroid therapy cannot be abruptly stopped?
   1. Higher steroid levels are needed during stress.
   2. Malignant hyperthermia will result.
   3. Malignant hypertension will occur.
   4. Respiratory failure will result.

8. The nurse is to provide preoperative teaching for a 74-year-old patient. Which of the following actions should the nurse take to improve learning?
   1. Sit in front of window in bright sunlight.
   2. Use small, white-on-black printed materials.
   3. Speak in a high tone.
   4. Eliminate background noise.

9. The nurse is caring for a postoperative patient. Which of the following complications would the nurse explain to the patient can be prevented with early postoperative ambulation?
   1. Increased peristalsis
   2. Coughing
   3. Pneumonia
   4. Wound healing

10. Which of the following actions should the nurse take to maintain patient safety when ambulating a patient for the first time postoperatively?
    1. Use one person to assist patient.
    2. Use two people to assist patient.
    3. Encourage patient to "dangle" self 1 hour before ambulation.
    4. Give narcotic 15 minutes before ambulation.

11. The nurse is caring for a patient with a bowel resection. Which of the following would indicate that the patient's gastrointestinal tract is resuming normal function?
    1. Firm abdomen
    2. Excessive thirst
    3. Presence of flatus
    4. Absent bowel sounds

12. The patient is dangling at the bedside and states, "Oh, my stomach is tearing open." Which of the following actions should the nurse immediately take when dehiscence occurs?
    1. Have patient sit upright in a chair.
    2. Slow IV fluids.
    3. Have patient lie down.
    4. Obtain a sterile suture set.

13. When the nurse is assisting the patient to use an incentive spirometer, which of the following actions by the patient indicates that the patient needs further teaching on how to use the spirometer?
    1. Taking two normal breaths before use
    2. Inhaling deeply to reach target
    3. Sitting upright before use
    4. Exhaling deeply to reach target

14. After surgery, the nurse notes that the patient's urine is dark amber and concentrated. Which of the following does the nurse understand may be the reason for this?
    1. The sympathetic nervous system saves fluid in response to stress of surgery.
    2. The sympathetic nervous system diureses fluid in response to stress of surgery.
    3. The parasympathetic nervous system saves fluid in response to stress of surgery.
    4. The parasympathetic nervous system diureses fluid in response to stress of surgery.

15. The patient develops a low-grade fever 18 hours postoperatively and has diminished breath sounds. Which of the following actions is most appropriate for the nurse to take to prevent complications? **Select all that apply.**
    1. Administer antibiotics.
    2. Encourage coughing and deep breathing.
    3. Administer acetaminophen (Tylenol).
    4. Decrease fluid intake.
    5. Ambulate patient as ordered.
    6. Monitor intake and output.

Nursing Care of Patients With Emergent Conditions and Disaster/Bioterrorism Response

13

VOCABULARY

Match the word with its definition.

1. _____ Skin scraped away because of injury.
2. _____ Disease caused by organism entering body through an open wound resulting in convulsions, muscle spasms, stiffness of the jaw, coma, and death.
3. _____ Insufficient intake of oxygen.
4. _____ Inadequate and progressively failing tissue perfusion that can result in cellular death.
5. _____ Irregular tear of the skin.
6. _____ Loss of water and electrolytes through heavy sweating, causing hypovolemia.
7. _____ Tearing away or crushing of body limbs.
8. _____ Frozen body parts that are white or yellow-white.
9. _____ A biological weapon that may occur in three forms: inhalational, cutaneous, and gastrointestinal.
10. _____ A biological weapon that can result in a severe febrile illness with hemoptysis as a classic sign.

1. Asphyxia
2. Tetanus
3. Abrasion
4. Laceration
5. Shock
6. Amputation
7. Heat exhaustion
8. Frostbite
9. Anthrax
10. Plague

PRINCIPLES FOR TREATING SHOCK

Indicate whether the statement is true or false and correct the false statement.

1. _____ Maintain an open airway and give oxygen as ordered.
2. _____ Control external bleeding by indirect pressure.
3. _____ Apply cooling blanket to cool patient.
4. _____ As possible, keep the patient supine.
5. _____ Take hourly vital signs.
6. _____ Give the patient oral fluids.
7. _____ Administer intravenous (IV) fluids as ordered.

SIGNS AND SYMPTOMS OF INCREASED INTRACRANIAL PRESSURE

Indicate whether the sign is an early sign or a late sign of increased intracranial pressure.

1. _____ Abnormal posturing
2. _____ Altered level of consciousness
3. _____ Amnesia
4. _____ Changes in respiratory pattern
5. _____ Changes in speech
6. _____ Decreased pulse rate
7. _____ Dilated nonreactive pupils
8. _____ Drowsiness
9. _____ Headache
10. _____ Nausea and vomiting
11. _____ Unresponsiveness
12. _____ Widening pulse pressure

1. Early sign
2. Late sign

ASSESSMENT OF MOTOR FUNCTION

Complete the table.

If the Patient Is Unable to:	The Lesion Is Above the Level of:
	C-5 to C-7
Extend and flex legs	
Flex foot, extend toes	
	S-3 to S-5

HYPERTHERMIA

Indicate whether the sign is an early sign or a late sign of hyperthermia caused by exposure to a hot environment.

1. _____ Core body temperature of 100.4° to 102.2°F (38°–39°C)
2. _____ Diaphoresis
3. _____ Hot, dry, flushed skin
4. _____ Hypotension
5. _____ Pulse rate more than 100
6. _____ Increasing body core temperature of 106°F (41°C) or more
7. _____ Cool, clammy skin
8. _____ Altered mental status
9. _____ Coma or seizures
10. _____ Dizziness

1. Early sign
2. Late sign

PRINCIPLES FOR DISASTER OR BIOTERRORISM RESPONSE

Fill in the blank.

1. A disaster _____ existing personnel, facilities, and equipment.

2. Hospitals activate _____ in a disaster.

3. In a disaster, off-duty staff members are _____, and noncritical patients are _____.

4. The emergency department serves as the _____ and _____ area.

5. Those treated first are the most _____ injured but who have the greatest chance for _____ recovery.

6. Disaster _____ are conducted on a regular basis.

7. You should be _____ with your _____ in a disaster.

8. Clinical illness from a biological weapon may differ from _____ infections.

CRITICAL THINKING

Read the case study and answer the questions.

Mr. Harvey, age 66, retired 1 year ago and made plans to travel with his wife. His wife unexpectedly died from a myocardial infarction 2 months ago. Mr. Harvey now lives alone. He has been withdrawn and rarely leaves the house since his wife's funeral. His son, Ted, who lives in another state, arrives for a weekend visit and is concerned about his father's behavior. Mr. Harvey has not bathed and is wearing soiled clothing. The refrigerator is bare, and he keeps the curtains drawn. He continually paces and says, "I want to die." Ted takes his father to the local emergency room.

1. Why might Mr. Harvey be exhibiting this behavior change?_____

_____

_____

_____

2. What symptoms of an acute psychiatric episode is Mr. Harvey exhibiting? _____

_____

_____

_____

3. Why should Mr. Harvey be referred for treatment?

_____

_____

_____

_____

4. What nursing diagnoses apply to Mr. Harvey? _____

_____

_____

_____

5. What nursing interventions are appropriate for Mr. Harvey initially? _____

_____

_____

_____

REVIEW QUESTIONS—CONTENT REVIEW

Choose the best answer unless directed otherwise.

1. For a patient who experiences anaphylactic shock after receiving a medication, which one of the following symptoms would the nurse anticipate?
   1. Chest pain
   2. Hot, dry skin
   3. Difficulty breathing
   4. Fever

2. The nurse is assessing a patient's extremity, which may be fractured. Which of the following is the nurse's purpose in checking capillary refill during the assessment?
   1. To evaluate arterial blood flow in an extremity
   2. To assess venous blood flow in an extremity
   3. To measure oxygen saturation of the blood
   4. To assess peripheral edema

3. During data collection, which of the following findings would indicate to the nurse that severe blood loss has occurred?
   1. Normal, bounding pulse
   2. Slow, strong pulse
   3. Rapid, thready pulse
   4. Slow, bounding pulse

REVIEW QUESTIONS—TEST PREPARATION

Choose the best answer unless directed otherwise.

4. Which of the following monitoring is a priority for the nurse when caring for a patient with botulism exposure?
   1. Gag reflex
   2. Pupil response
   3. Corneal reflex
   4. Babinski's response

5. The nurse anticipates that treatment for an unconscious patient who has ingested 50 tablets of alprazolam (Xanax), a noncaustic substance, might include which of the following?
   1. Administering an antiemetic
   2. Administering activated charcoal
   3. Forced vomiting
   4. Forcing fluids

6. The nurse is planning care for a patient who has hyperthermia. Which of the following indicates that treatment is effective?
   1. Core body temperature less than 94°F (34.4°C)
   2. Patient alert and oriented
   3. Skin cool and moist to touch
   4. Core body temperature greater than 101°F (38.3°C)

7. The health care provider orders haloperidol (Haldol) 3 mg intramuscularly for a patient who is experiencing a psychiatric crisis. Haloperidol 5 mg/mL is available. How many milliliters should the nurse give?
   1. 0.3 mL
   2. 0.5 mL
   3. 0.6 mL
   4. 1.3 mL

8. The nurse is collecting data on a patient with a large bleeding laceration. Which of the following requires immediate intervention by the nurse?
   1. Thready pulse at 116
   2. Strong pulse at 84
   3. Weak pulse at 56
   4. Bounding pulse at 66

9. The nurse is admitting a trauma patient to the emergency department. Place in order of priority the areas on which data are collected as the nurse performs the primary survey. Use all options.
   1. Circulation
   2. Breathing
   3. Airway
   4. Disability

10. The nurse is caring for a patient who is bleeding from the radial artery. The nurse is applying direct pressure to the radial artery and has elevated the arm, but the wound continues to bleed. Which of the following actions should the nurse take now?
    1. Apply pressure to the carotid artery.
    2. Apply pressure to the brachial artery.
    3. Apply pressure to the femoral artery.
    4. Apply pressure to the temporal artery.

11. The nurse is caring for a patient with a painful rash on the face and forearms who is febrile. Which of the following items is important for the nurse who is unvaccinated to use while providing care to the patient? **Select all that apply.**
    1. Mask
    2. Gown
    3. Gloves
    4. Fit-tested N95 respirator
    5. Shoe covers
    6. Hair net

unit THREE

Understanding Life Span Influences on Health and Illness

CHECKLIST FOR LEARNING SUCCESS

Influences on Health and Illness

- ❏ Health, wellness, illness
- ❏ Nurse's role in supporting and promoting wellness
- ❏ Young adult
- ❏ Middle-aged adult
- ❏ Older adult
- ❏ Chronic illness
- ❏ Nursing care

Nursing Care of Older Adult Patients

- ❏ Physiological aging changes
- ❏ Cognitive and psychological aging changes
- ❏ Health promotion for older patients
- ❏ Nursing implications for older patients

Nursing Care of Patients at Home

- ❏ Introduction to home health nursing
- ❏ History of home health nursing
- ❏ Home health eligibility
- ❏ Home health care team
- ❏ Transition from hospital-based nursing to home health care
- ❏ The role of the LPN/LVN in home health
- ❏ Steps in the home health visit
- ❏ Nursing process: the home health patient
- ❏ Other forms of home health nursing

Nursing Care of Patients at the End of Life

- ❏ Identifying impending death
- ❏ Advance directive
- ❏ Living wills
- ❏ Durable medical power of attorney
- ❏ End-of-life choices
- ❏ Communicating with dying patients
- ❏ The dying process
- ❏ Grieving

14

Developmental Considerations in the Nursing Care of Adults

VOCABULARY

Unscramble the word that fits the definition.

1. Short-term intermittent rest provided to caregivers—*serptei crea* _____
2. Perception that one's own actions will not affect an outcome—*wporelsesesns* _____
3. Condition of long duration—*rhcnoic* _____
4. Life principles that pervade one's being—*sitrpiauilty* _____
5. State in which person sees no alternatives or choices—*pohelesnsses* _____
6. A certain time frame during one's life containing tasks an individual needs to accomplish for high-level wellness—*evdlepoemnatl taseg* _____

CHRONIC ILLNESS AND THE OLDER ADULT

Find and correct the eight errors.

Older adults constitute one of the smallest age groups living with chronic illness. Older adult spouses or older family members rarely have to care for a chronically ill family member. Children of older adults who themselves are reaching their 40s are being expected to care for their parents. These older adult caregivers do not experience chronic illness themselves. For older adult spouses, it is usually the less ill spouse who provides care to the other spouse. The older adult family unit is at great risk for ineffective coping or further development of health problems. Nurses should assess ill members of the older adult family to ensure that their health needs are being met.

Older adults are not concerned about becoming dependent and a burden to others. They may become depressed and give up hope if they feel that they are a burden. Establishing long-term goals or self-care activities that allow them to participate or have small successes are important nursing actions that can decrease their self-esteem.

CRITICAL THINKING

Read the case study and answer the questions.

Mrs. Martin is hospitalized for an exacerbation of her multiple sclerosis. She tells the nurse she is tired of being ill and is not getting any better. She says, "When I am in the hospital, I cannot attend church, which is my only enjoyment." Later in the day, Mrs. Martin is tearful and withdrawn when the nurse makes rounds.

1. What further data collection should the nurse obtain to identify Mrs. Martin's patient-centered needs? _____

   _____

   _____

2. What possible nursing diagnoses would be appropriate for Mrs. Martin? _____

   _____

   _____

3. What patient-centered care interventions could the nurse use to assist Mrs. Martin in meeting her wish to attend church? _____

_____

_____

4. How would the nurse know that Mrs. Martin's goal has been met? _____

_____

REVIEW QUESTIONS—CONTENT REVIEW

Choose the best answer unless directed otherwise.

1. The nurse is caring for a 72-year-old patient. As the nurse identifies the patient's developmental stage, which of the following of Erikson's developmental stages would the nurse expect the patient to be in?
   1. Generativity versus self-absorption
   2. Identity versus role confusion
   3. Intimacy versus isolation
   4. Integrity versus despair

2. The nurse is assessing the family of a patient with dementia. Which of the following findings would the nurse anticipate finding for caregivers of patients who are chronically ill when respite care is not available?
   1. Personal time increases.
   2. Rest time increases.
   3. Financial costs increase.
   4. Stress levels increase.

3. The nurse is planning care for a patient with heart failure. Which of the following is a health promotion method for the nurse to use that is helpful for the patient who is chronically ill?
   1. Making the choices for the patient
   2. Setting the goals for the family
   3. Setting the goals for the patient
   4. Allowing the patient to make informed decisions

4. The nurse is assigned to care for a group of patients with the following conditions. Which of these does the nurse understand is an example of a chronic illness to plan patient-centered care?
   1. Arthritis
   2. Bowel obstruction
   3. Cellulitis
   4. Peritonitis

5. The nurse is caring for a patient with a chronic illness. The nurse would evaluate the patient as fulfilling a primary task that patients who are chronically ill need to perform if the patient reported doing which of these actions?
   1. Being willing and able to carry out the medical regimen
   2. Reducing social activities to compensate for limitations
   3. Learning how to play the sick role
   4. Refusing to accept negative changes

REVIEW QUESTIONS—TEST PREPARATION

Choose the best answer unless directed otherwise.

6. The nurse is assigned to care for a group of patients. Which of these does the nurse understand is an example of a congenital chronic illness to plan patient-centered care? **Select all that apply.**
   1. Head injury
   2. Malabsorption syndrome
   3. Chronic obstructive pulmonary disease
   4. Arthritis
   5. Cystic fibrosis
   6. Spina bifida

7. The nurse is developing a plan of care for a patient, age 68, focusing on preventive health care. While planning this care, the nurse understands that aging processes are most affected by which of the following factors?
   1. Stress management
   2. Financial issues
   3. Age at retirement
   4. Hobbies

8. A patient, age 64, is active and wants to learn health promotion interventions. Which of the following actions by the nurse supports the patient's desire for self-health promotion?
   1. Assign responsibilities for the patient's care to family members.
   2. Select a family physician for the patient.
   3. List health care activities for the patient to carry out.
   4. Ask the patient to select desired health care activities.

9. The home care nurse is caring for a patient with emphysema who seems depressed. Which of the following nursing interventions increases the patient's participation in self-care and assists with improving the patient's depression?
   1. Being a caretaker instead of a partner
   2. Assisting the patient rather than doing everything for the patient
   3. Performing activities of daily living for the patient instead of empowering the patient
   4. Doing everything for the patient instead of assisting the patient

10. The nurse is caring for a patient who is recovering from a stroke. Which of the following nursing interventions during rehabilitation will MOST increase the patient's self-esteem?
    1. Offering praise for small patient efforts
    2. Offering praise for major patient efforts
    3. Performing activities of daily living for the patient
    4. Assisting patient at first sign of difficulty with activities of daily living

11. The nurse is caring for a patient who is secluded and sad. Which of the following nursing actions might be MOST helpful for psychosocial intervention for the patient who is withdrawn, depressed, or tense because of isolation resulting from a chronic illness?
    1. Avoiding the use of humor
    2. Reading comics or jokes from magazines
    3. Maintaining a serious demeanor
    4. Limiting conversation to a minimum

12. The nurse is caring for a patient who is chronically ill. In contributing to the plan of care for the patient who is chronically ill, which of the following is an appropriate nursing intervention designed to empower the patient?
    1. Provide educational information.
    2. Limit visiting hours for family members.
    3. Ask family members to provide care.
    4. Set goals for the patient and family.

13. The nurse is caring for a patient with Huntington's disease. The family asks what the cause of the illness is. Which of the following responses is most appropriate by the nurse?
    1. "Huntington's disease is a genetic disorder; the family may want to consider genetic testing."
    2. "Huntington's disease is a congenital disorder that developed in the womb."
    3. "Huntington's disease is an acquired disorder caused by smoking."
    4. "Huntington's disease is common among people over age 65, but the cause is unknown."

Nursing Care of Older Adult Patients

15

VOCABULARY

Fill in the blank with the word for the definition.

1. _____ Behaviors that are performed in the care and maintenance of self and surroundings

2. _____ Irregular heart rhythm

3. _____ Opacity of the lens of the eye, its capsule, or both

4. _____ State of feeling or mind

5. _____ Accidental drawing of foreign substances into the airway

6. _____ Collection of excess fluid in body tissues

7. _____ A group of eye diseases characterized by increased intraocular pressure

8. _____ The act or process of coughing up materials from the air passageways leading to the lungs

9. _____ A condition of sluggish or difficult bowel action/evacuation

10. _____ The body's attempts to maintain a balance whenever a change occurs

11. _____ Abnormal accumulation of fibrosis connective tissue in skin, muscle, or joint capsule that prevents normal mobility

12. _____ An open sore or lesion of the skin that develops because of prolonged pressure against an area

13. _____ Excessive urination at night

14. _____ External variables that determine the occurrence and rate of structural and functional declines in the human body over time

15. _____ Age-related breakdown of the macular area of the retina of the eye, disrupting central vision

16. _____ A condition in which there is a reduction in the mass of bone per unit volume

17. _____ None or minimal stimulation of senses that creates potential for maladaptive coping

18. _____ Highest level of patient activity considering the patient's condition

19. _____ A process to orient a person to names, dates, time, and other pertinent information through use of repeating messages

20. _____ Excessive stimulation of the senses that creates the potential for maladaptive coping

AGING CHANGES

Match the aging change with the effect of the change.

1. _____ Increased conduction time	1. Heart rate slows, unable to increase quickly
2. _____ Decreased blood vessel elasticity	2. Less oxygen delivered to tissues
3. _____ Leg veins dilate, valves become less efficient	3. Increased blood pressure and cardiac workload
4. _____ Basal metabolic rate slows	4. Poor heart oxygenation
5. _____ Decreased cardiac output	5. Varicose veins, fluid accumulation in tissues
6. _____ Decreased insulin release	6. Possible weight gain
7. _____ Irregular heartbeats	7. Decreased ability to respond to stress
8. _____ Altered adrenal hormone production	8. Hyperglycemia
9. _____ Decreased gag reflex	9. Appetite may be reduced
10. _____ Decreased peristalsis	10. Dry mouth, altered taste
11. _____ Reduced liver enzymes	11. Increased aspiration risk
12. _____ Decreased saliva	12. Frequency of urination
13. _____ Delayed gastric emptying	13. Reduced drug metabolism/detoxification
14. _____ Decreased bladder size and tone, changes from pear to funnel shaped	14. Reduced appetite, constipation
15. _____ Decreased kidney concentrating ability	15. Nocturia
16. _____ Less sodium saved	16. Risk of dehydration
17. _____ Reduced renal blood flow	17. Decreased renal clearance of all medications
18. _____ Decreased immune function	18. Greater infection and cancer risk
19. _____ Body content water loss	19. Slower healing process
20. _____ Decreased sebaceous/sweat gland	20. Dryness of the skin
21. _____ Reduced cell replacement	21. Decreased temperature regulation
22. _____ Muscle responses slowed	22. Response time increased
23. _____ Decreased brain blood flow	23. Short-term memory loss
24. _____ Less vaginal lubrication	24. Risk of injury, burns
25. _____ Decreased sensation	25. Dyspnea with activity
26. _____ Decreased lung capacity	26. Painful intercourse

COMMUNICATING WITH PEOPLE WHO HAVE HEARING IMPAIRMENTS

Indicate whether the statement is true or false and correct false statements.

1. _____ Ensure that hearing aids are turned on and have working batteries.
2. _____ The speaker should turn to the side so the speaker's profile is visible to patient.
3. _____ Speak toward the patient's impaired side of hearing.
4. _____ Speak in a clear, moderate-volume, low-pitched tone.
5. _____ Do not shout because doing so distorts sounds.
6. _____ Recognize that high-frequency tones and consonant sounds are lost last—s, z, sh, ch, d, g.
7. _____ Eliminate background noise because it distorts sounds.

MEDICATIONS

Find the six errors and correct them.

Older patients are less susceptible to drug-induced illness and adverse medication side effects for various reasons. They take few medicines for the one chronic illness that they have. Different medications interact and produce side effects that can be dangerous. Over-the-counter medicines that older patients take, as well as the self-prescribed extracts, elixirs, herbal teas, cultural healing substances, and other home remedies commonly used by individuals of their age cohort do not influence other medications.

If an older patient crushes a large enteric-coated pill so it can be taken in food and is easily swallowed, it enhances the enteric protection and can inadvertently cause damage to the stomach and intestinal system. Some patients unintentionally skip prescribed doses in an effort to save money. When prescribed doses are not being taken as expected, problems do not clear up as quickly, and new problems may result. The nurse should educate the older patient and the patient's family. Patients need to know what each prescribed pill is for, when it is prescribed to be taken, and how it should be taken.

CRITICAL THINKING

Read the following case study and answer the questions. This is a values clarification exercise.

While making 2200 rounds in the extended care facility, the nurse looks into Mr. B's room to find Mr. B and a female resident from down the hall together, sleeping soundly in Mr. B's bed with the side rails up. Mr. B and the female resident are both 63 years of age. Mr. S, who is Mr. B's roommate, is sound asleep alone in his own bed.

1. What are your initial feelings about this situation?

_____

_____

_____

2. What influences your feelings? _____

_____

_____

3. What is the first thing that you would do after this discovery? _____

_____

_____

4. What issues should you consider before making a decision? _____

_____

_____

5. How will you interact with these patients in the future?

_____

_____

_____

REVIEW QUESTIONS—CONTENT REVIEW

Choose the best answer unless directed otherwise.

1. The nurse understands that wax buildup in an older patient's ears can cause which type of hearing loss?
   1. Sensorineural
   2. Bone conduction
   3. Perceptive
   4. Neural

2. The nurse understands that which of the following factors is most often the cause of sexual dysfunction for older people?
   1. Physical factors
   2. Psychological factors
   3. Social factors
   4. Environmental factors

3. Which of the following actions should be taken to help an older person prevent osteoporosis?
   1. Decrease dietary intake of calcium.
   2. Encourage regular exercise.
   3. Increase dietary intake of salt.
   4. Increase dietary protein intake.

REVIEW QUESTIONS—TEST PREPARATION

Choose the best answer unless directed otherwise.

4. A 72-year-old patient has been seeing a doctor for treatment of glaucoma for the past 5 years. Which of the following symptoms does the nurse expect the patient to relate when discussing the symptoms?
   1. Headaches more severe in the evening
   2. Blurred vision when attempting to focus
   3. Morning headaches that disappear after rising
   4. Increased sensitivity to light in the early morning

5. As the nurse performs an oral assessment on an 84-year-old patient, which of the following is an expected finding within the patient's mouth caused by advancing age?
   1. Loss of teeth
   2. Hardness of the gums
   3. Increased production of saliva
   4. Decreased taste sensitivity for salt

6. As the nurse collects data on a 79-year-old patient, which of the following does the nurse recognize as an aging change in the cardiovascular system?
   1. Increased cardiac output
   2. Increased peripheral vascular resistance
   3. Increased resting heart rate
   4. Increased cardiac reserve

7. Which of the following does the nurse understand is the rationale for dangling a 70-year-old patient at the bedside before helping the patient to stand upright?
   1. To provide a heightened awareness of body position
   2. To accommodate a less efficient circulatory system
   3. To strengthen legs
   4. To reduce anxiety about getting up

8. As the nurse provides care to an 80-year-old patient with an intravenous (IV) infusion, the nurse understands that it is essential for older patients who are receiving IV fluids to be monitored closely to prevent which of the following?
   1. Circulatory distress
   2. Dislodging of the IV
   3. Venous distention
   4. Increased urinary output

9. The nurse is talking with a patient who is hard of hearing and is having the most difficulty with high-pitched tones. To increase the patient's hearing, which of the following should the nurse do when speaking with the patient?
   1. Speak slowly with emphasis on important words.
   2. Double the voice volume.
   3. Whisper responses in proximity to the patient's ear.
   4. Use a modulated voice and talk normally in either ear.

10. A nurse is working in an extended care facility. Which of the following nursing behaviors demonstrates the nurse's respect for the older patient's sexuality?
    1. Providing privacy time for a patient by enclosing the bed with the curtain and ensuring that the patient is undisturbed for an hour
    2. Entering a patient's room without knocking when a visitor is present
    3. Walking in on a patient and visitor during an embrace to prepare medications
    4. Changing the subject when a patient expresses feelings toward a friend

11. A nurse caring for a number of older clients on a medical unit recognizes that which of the following individuals would be at highest risk for using a prescription medication considered inappropriate?
    1. A 60-year-old college professor recently diagnosed with diabetes admitted with cellulitis.
    2. A 72-year-old high school dropout who suffered double below-the-knee amputations in the Korean War admitted with a decubitus ulcer.
    3. A 76-year-old retired lawyer with a history of hypertension and chronic renal failure admitted for dehydration.
    4. An 81-year-old retired teacher with a history of colorectal cancer admitted for a colonoscopy.

Nursing Care of Patients at Home

16

VOCABULARY

Match the term to the correct definition.

1. _____ Autonomous
2. _____ Case management
3. _____ Certified
4. _____ Collaborative care
5. _____ Community resources
6. _____ Homebound
7. _____ Private duty
8. _____ Respite care
9. _____ Skilled nursing
10. _____ Start of care

1. Care that can only be delivered by a licensed professional nurse
2. Occurs when a patient is unable to leave his or her home to obtain necessary health services
3. To work together to achieve a goal
4. Coordinates care among patient, health care provider, and caregivers
5. A health care provider's order that allows home health services to care for a patient for 60 days
6. To work independently
7. Available to a home health patient to improve his or her quality of care; usually coordinated by a social service worker
8. Scheduled care to assist the patient with personnel and homemaking needs
9. Begins on the first day of nursing services
10. Provides family members and caregivers time to take care of themselves

HOME HEALTH SERVICES

Match the home health services/role to the appropriate definition.

1. _____ Social services
2. _____ Physical therapy
3. _____ Occupational therapy
4. _____ Registered nurse
5. _____ Certified nursing assistant
6. _____ Licensed practical nurse/licensed vocational nurse (LPN/LVN)
7. _____ Speech therapist
8. _____ Health care provider

1. Assists the patient with activities of daily living (ADLs)
2. Develops the plan of care and manages the care of the patient during home health services
3. Assists the patient with developing independence with ADLs
4. Assists the patient with access to community resources
5. Assists the patient with strength and gait training
6. Works with language, speech, swallowing
7. Team leader
8. Makes home visits and performs skilled nursing care.

CRITICAL THINKING

Read the following case study and answer the questions.

Mrs. Thompson was just discharged from the hospital after an exacerbation of her respiratory disease. Her health history includes chronic obstructive pulmonary disease (COPD), type 2 diabetes, and coronary artery disease (CAD). She is receiving O_2 therapy at 2 L/minute via nasal cannula. She has a skin tear on her right lower extremity requiring dressing changes every other day for 4 weeks. The physician increased her heart medications to include a beta blocker for heart rate control.

Mrs. Thompson lives alone and has verbalized to the registered nurse (RN), on admission, that it is difficult for her to prepare meals and "get around the house." She has one married daughter who lives locally and works full time.

1. How often will Mrs. Thompson require skilled nursing services? _____

_____

_____

2. What services will the home health nurse be performing?

_____

_____

_____

3. What are some safety considerations for Mrs. Thompson?

_____

_____

4. Would Mrs. Thompson benefit from any other home health services? _____

_____

_____

REVIEW QUESTIONS—CONTENT REVIEW

Choose the best answer unless directed otherwise.

1. Which of the following nursing leaders demonstrated the impact nurses can have with the care and improvement of patients in the home?
   1. Florence Nightingale
   2. Clara Barton
   3. Lillian Wald
   4. Jean Watson

2. A patient has just been discharged from the hospital after open heart surgery. The patient's spouse is the primary caregiver and confides that handling all of the finances, the patient's complex medication regime, assistance with ADLs, and general household management is a concern. Which of the following would be an appropriate nursing diagnosis for the patient's spouse?
   1. Ineffective Coping
   2. Powerlessness
   3. Ineffective Health Maintenance
   4. Risk for Caregiver Role Strain

3. When providing care to a patient in the patient's home, the nurse understands that which of the following persons is in control of the home care environment?
   1. Family
   2. Health care provider
   3. Nurse
   4. Patient

REVIEW QUESTIONS—TEST PREPARATION

Choose the best answer unless directed otherwise.

4. The nurse is making a first-time visit to a patient at home. Which of the following techniques could the home health nurse use to develop trust with the patient?
   1. Review patient's history to plan patient needs before visit.
   2. Call the night before the visit to set a time for the visit.
   3. Acknowledge patient's fears that are expressed.
   4. Discuss treatment plans with the patient only.

5. The nurse collects safety data on an initial visit to the home of a patient who has returned home from the hospital and has an infected abdominal wound requiring dressing changes. Which of the following interventions should the nurse include in the plan of care to promote safety in the home? **Select all that apply.**
   1. Explain to the patient never to get out of bed without assistance.
   2. Instruct a family member to be available at all times to assist with ambulation.
   3. Clean the patient's home each visit to maintain asepsis.
   4. Instruct the family to remove all scatter rugs.
   5. Ask family to install handrails in the hallway for ambulation.
   6. Clear walkways of all clutter.

6. The nurse arrives at a patient's home. Which of the following interventions performed by the nurse would demonstrate understanding of the importance of following infection control principles in the home?
   1. Setting the nurse's home health bag on the floor
   2. Cleaning supplies after each home health visit
   3. Hand washing in the patient's kitchen sink
   4. Using dressing supplies sitting opened on a table

7. The nurse is to give a patient morphine 8 mg intramuscular for pain. The nurse has available 10 mg of morphine/mL. How many mL will the nurse give?
   _____ mL

8. The nurse is making a home visit to a 68-year-old patient and is reinforcing medication teaching that was done in the hospital setting. The nurse understands that the teaching will be more effective with which of the following techniques? **Select all that apply.**
   1. Provide a long teaching session.
   2. Include a support person.
   3. Make instructions simple.
   4. Provide demonstration.
   5. Repeat instructions often.

9. The LPN is visiting a patient to check blood glucose and administer insulin. As the LPN obtains the insulin from the refrigerator where the patient stores it, the LPN observes that dirty dishes are stacked in the kitchen sink, and there is only a moldy opened can of soup, a sandwich, and cat food in the refrigerator. Which of the following actions should the LPN take regarding the visit findings?
   1. Inform the RN of the moldy and sparse food.
   2. Tell the patient to wash the dishes.
   3. Notify the RN that the patient is eating cat food.
   4. Wash the dirty dishes.

10. Which of the following could the nurse do to prepare for a home health visit and ensure that it is a safe and effective visit? **Select all that apply.**
    1. Give the patient a time range for arrival.
    2. Provide an exact time for arrival.
    3. Obtain driving directions to the patient's home.
    4. Park in the patient's driveway.
    5. Keep gas tank filled.
    6. Carry a whistle.

11. The nurse is visiting an 89-year-old woman in the home to assess the need for skilled nursing care after a fall resulting in a broken collarbone. Which of the following should be included in the nurse's initial visit? **Select all that apply.**
    1. Identify fall risks in the home environment.
    2. Observe the patient perform activities of daily living.
    3. Collect baseline vital signs.
    4. Obtain a urine sample for culture and sensitivity.
    5. Review patient medications and schedule.

17

Nursing Care of Patients at the End of Life

VOCABULARY

Fill in the blank.

1. Part of an advance directive is a document instructing caregivers in patients' medical preferences at end of life, called a _____.

2. A _____ document specifies who can make decisions for a patient when the patient can no longer make decisions.

3. Patients qualify for _____ care when their prognosis is 6 months or less.

4. Care of the body after death is called _____ _____.

5. The nurse who communicates patients' and families' wishes to the health team is acting as a patient _____.

TRUE OR FALSE?

Indicate whether the statement is true or false and correct false statements.

1. _____ Older adult patients usually gain weight while undergoing treatment in a hospital.

2. _____ Only a few health insurance companies provide a hospice benefit.

3. _____ Insomnia, headaches, and fatigue can be a sign of grief in nurses.

4. _____ Dehydration in dying patients causes endorphins to be released that will enhance comfort.

5. _____ Patients who live longer than 6 months while on hospice will be discharged from the hospice program.

6. _____ Terminal illness is experienced by the whole family.

7. _____ To improve the chance of success for patients receiving cardiopulmonary resuscitation (CPR) at the time of cardiac arrest, CPR must be started within 8 minutes.

8. _____ One benefit of withholding artificial fluids in patients who are actively dying is fewer pharyngeal and lung secretions.

9. _____ Eighty percent of communication with terminal patients and their families is nonverbal.

10. _____ Confusion and agitation are two common indicators that older adult patients are approaching the end of life.

CRITICAL THINKING

Read the following case study and answer the questions.

Your patient, Mrs. Brown, is actively dying from end-stage lung cancer. List at least two nursing interventions that may be helpful to treat each symptom she is experiencing:

1. Dyspnea _____

_____

_____

2. Bowel and bladder incontinence _____

_____

_____

3. Copious oral secretions _____

_____

_____

4. Body temperature changes _____

_____

_____

5. Restlessness _____

_____

_____

REVIEW QUESTIONS—CONTENT REVIEW

Choose the best answer unless directed otherwise.

1. Research on patients with dementia who received tube feedings revealed which of the following risks?
   1. The risk of aspiration was decreased.
   2. The risk of aspiration was increased.
   3. The patients gained excess weight.
   4. Pressure ulcers healed more quickly.

2. What question can be most effective in finding out the patient's understanding of the severity of the illness he or she is experiencing?
   1. "How do you feel about your illness?"
   2. "How is your family coping with your illness?"
   3. "What has the doctor told you about your illness?"
   4. "What would you like to do about your illness?"

3. A dying patient's family members are upset and crying. Which action by the nurse will best help the family?
   1. Sustain eye contact and encourage them to talk about their concerns.
   2. Ask them to speak quietly so as not to disturb the other patients.
   3. Tell them for the sake of their loved one, they need to compose themselves.
   4. Move them to another room away from the patient.

REVIEW QUESTIONS—TEST PREPARATION

Choose the best answer unless directed otherwise.

4. A family member asks why a dying patient is receiving morphine when the patient doesn't appear to be in any pain. Which response by the nurse is best?
   1. "Morphine helps make patients less aware of their surroundings."
   2. "Morphine helps patients breathe more comfortably."
   3. "Morphine helps keep body temperature under control."
   4. "Morphine helps patients sleep."

5. A patient has just been pronounced dead. What is the first action the nurse should take?
   1. Contact the nursing supervisor.
   2. Remove the patient's tubes and create a clean, peaceful impression for the family.
   3. Make sure the patient gets to the funeral home within 12 hours for embalming.
   4. Move the patient out of the hospital room to the morgue.

6. A dying patient appears confused and keeps saying he sees his wife who died 10 years earlier. The family appears upset by this. What teaching should the nurse provide?
   1. Teach them to redirect the patient and gently remind him that his wife died long ago.
   2. Explain that this happens because of the medications that the patient is receiving.
   3. Explain that this is a common occurrence and encourage them to allow him to talk about his experience.
   4. Explain that this can occur when the brain is deprived of oxygen and then get an order for oxygen if the patient does not already have it.

7. An older patient with chronic disease is very weak and chokes when attempting to eat. The patient's daughter is upset and wants a feeding tube inserted. The physician has told her that the patient is dying and that a tube will not prolong life. The daughter is now crying in the hallway. Which response by the nurse is best?
   1. Reiterate what the doctor said about the patient not living any longer with a tube.
   2. Tell the daughter that a tube is uncomfortable for the patient.
   3. Tell the daughter the staff will feed him more slowly to prevent choking.
   4. Acknowledge how hard this is for her, as she has taken such good care of feeding the patient throughout the illness.

8. A patient being discharged from the hospital has decided she does not want to be resuscitated should she experience a cardiopulmonary arrest. Which of the following documents should the nurse assist the patient to complete?
   1. Living will
   2. Advance medical directive
   3. Durable power of attorney
   4. Physician orders for life-sustaining treatments (POLST)

9. The family of a patient who is terminally ill asks a nurse if they may bathe their loved one after death, in keeping with their cultural traditions. Which response is best?
   1. "You should concentrate on the time you have left together."
   2. "Your cultural traditions are important and will be supported by our staff."
   3. "Our staff will make sure the patient is clean and bathed."
   4. "That won't be necessary, because the funeral home takes care of bathing the patient."

10. The family members of a patient with terminal cancer have agreed to stop aggressive treatment and begin comfort measures only. Which of the following statements would the nurse include in a discussion of specific decisions? **Select all that apply.**
    1. "Withholding artificial hydration can make breathing more comfortable."
    2. "Pain may be reduced if artificial hydration is stopped because tumor swelling is decreased."
    3. "If the intravenous fluids are stopped, the patient's body will stop making endorphins."
    4. "Research indicates that tube feeding in people dying of cancer is not beneficial."
    5. "Patients who are not fed often say they are hungry as they are dying."

unit FOUR

Understanding the Immune System

CHECKLIST FOR LEARNING SUCCESS

Review of Anatomy and Physiology and Aging Changes	Major Disorders	Nursing Assessment	Diagnostic Tests	Interventions	Common Medications
❑ Immune:	❑ Immune:	❑ Medical history	❑ Blood studies	❑ Immunotherapy	❑ Antihistamines
❑ Antigens	❑ Allergic rhinitis	❑ Physical examination	❑ Radiographic tests	❑ Medications	❑ Antiretrovirals
❑ Lymphocytes	❑ Atopic dermatitis		❑ Biopsies	❑ Surgical management	❑ Corticosteroids
❑ Antibodies	❑ Anaphylaxis		❑ Skin tests	❑ Monoclonal Antibodies	❑ Epinephrine
❑ Mechanisms of immunity	❑ Urticaria		❑ Gene testing	❑ Recombinant DNA technology	❑ Fusion inhibitors
❑ Types of immunity	❑ Angioedema				❑ Immunosuppressives
❑ Aging effects	❑ Hemolytic transfusion reaction				❑ Immunoglobulin
	❑ Serum sickness				❑ Integrase inhibitors
	❑ Contact dermatitis				❑ Nonnucleoside analogue reverse transcriptase inhibitors
	❑ Transplant rejection				
	❑ Pernicious anemia				❑ Nucleoside analogue reverse transcriptase inhibitors
	❑ Idiopathic autoimmune hemolytic anemia				
	❑ Hashimoto's thyroiditis				❑ Nucleotide analogue reverse transcriptase inhibitors
	❑ Ankylosing spondylitis				
	❑ Lupus erythematosus				❑ Protease inhibitors
	❑ Hypogammaglobulinemia				❑ Ribonucleotide reductase inhibitors
	❑ Human immunodeficiency virus (HIV)				❑ Rho (D) immune globulin (RhoGAM)
	❑ Acquired immune deficiency syndrome (AIDS)				❑ Thyroxine
					❑ Vitamin B_{12}

18

Immune System Function, Assessment, and Therapeutic Measures

STRUCTURES OF THE IMMUNE SYSTEM

Label the following structures.

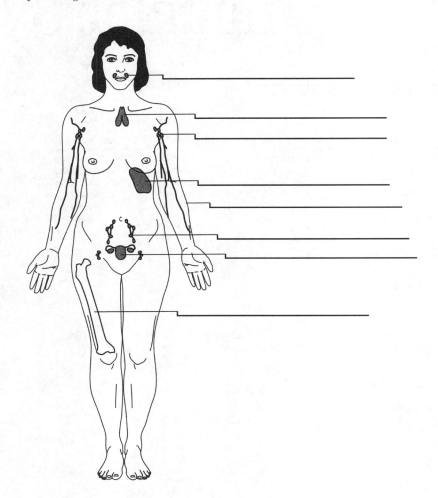

IMMUNE SYSTEM CELLS

Match each cell of the immune system with the correct description.

1. _____ Memory cells
2. _____ Helper T cells
3. _____ Cytotoxic T cells
4. _____ Plasma cells
5. _____ Suppressor T cells
6. _____ Macrophages
7. _____ B cells

1. Phagocytize pathogens labeled with antibodies
2. Produce antibodies
3. Limit the immune response once the pathogen has been destroyed
4. Initiate a rapid immune response if the pathogen reenters the body
5. Destroy cells directly by lysing their membranes
6. May become plasma cells or memory cells
7. Participate in antigen recognition and activate B cells

ANTIBODIES

Name the proper class of antibodies for each of these functions.

1. Found in mucous membrane secretions: _____
2. Provides long-term immunity: _____
3. Form the receptors on B cells: _____
4. Important in allergic reactions: _____
5. Cross the placenta to fetal circulation: _____
6. Found in breast milk: _____
7. The first antibody produced in an infection: _____

VOCABULARY

Fill in the blank.

1. _____ are chemical markers that identify cells or molecules.
2. _____ is the ability to destroy pathogens or other foreign material and to prevent further cases of certain infectious diseases.
3. _____, _____, and _____ are the three types of lymphocytes.
4. _____ mature in the thymus gland.
5. Antibodies are also called _____.
6. _____ immunity is the type of immunity that involves only T cells.
7. _____ immunity is the type of immunity in which a person has recovered from a disease and now has antibodies and memory cells specific for that pathogen.
8. The immunoglobulin _____ provides long-term immunity following recovery from an illness.
9. Lymph node enlargement with tenderness is usually indicative of _____.
10. The _____ of a white blood cell differential are increased in bacterial infections.

IMMUNE SYSTEM

Match the word with the definition.

1. _____ Allergy shots
2. _____ Tests for antibodies to human immunodeficiency virus (HIV), used as a screening test
3. _____ Important in allergic reactions and attaches to mast cells
4. _____ Swelling around the eyes
5. _____ A test done to confirm a diagnosis, determine a prognosis, or evaluate effectiveness of treatment
6. _____ Found in secretions of all mucous membranes
7. _____ Itching
8. _____ An abnormal protein found in plasma during an acute inflammatory process

1. Periorbital edema
2. Biopsies
3. Pruritus
4. Enzyme-linked immunosorbent assay
5. IgE
6. C-reactive protein
7. Immunotherapy
8. IgA

DATA COLLECTION—HISTORY

Find and correct the 12 errors.

Demographic Data

The patient's age, gender, race, and ethnic background are important. Systemic lupus erythematosus affects men eight times more frequently than women. The patient's place of birth gives insight into ethnic ties. Where the patient has lived and does live may shed light on the current illness. The patient's occupation, such as that of a coal miner, may contribute to gastrointestinal symptoms.

Rare signs and symptoms found with immune system disorders include fever, fatigue, joint pain, swollen glands, weight gain, and skin rash.

History

Food, medication, and environmental allergies should include those that the patient experiences and those present in the family history. With a family history, a previous exposure to a substance is required before a severe reaction occurs. Conditions such as allergic rhinitis, systemic lupus erythematosus, ankylosing spondylitis, and asthma are thought to be either familial or have a congenital predisposition. If the patient's thymus gland has been removed (thymectomy), B-cell production may be altered. Corticosteroids and immunosuppressants enhance the immune response. The patient's lifestyle may place the patient at low risk for contracting the human immunodeficiency virus. The patient's diet and usage of vitamins give insight into the depletion of the immune system. Stress (environmental, physical, and psychological) can enhance immune system function.

CRITICAL THINKING

Read the following case study and answer the questions.

David Case, age 29, is visiting his health care provider because he has been extremely fatigued for several months and now has swollen lymph nodes in his neck. On palpation, the area feels enlarged, nontender, hard, and fixed.

1. What categories of data collection should the nurse obtain? _____
   _____
   _____
   _____

2. What might the palpation findings indicate?
   _____
   _____
   _____
   _____

3. What categories of data collection would be important to explore in detail? _____
   _____
   _____
   _____

REVIEW QUESTIONS—CONTENT REVIEW

Choose the best answer unless directed otherwise.

1. A baby is born temporarily immune to the diseases to which the mother is immune. The nurse would explain this to the mother as being which of the following types of immunity?
   1. Naturally acquired passive immunity
   2. Artificially acquired passive immunity
   3. Naturally acquired active immunity
   4. Artificially acquired active immunity

2. Immunity to a disease after recovery is possible because the first exposure to the pathogen has stimulated the formation of which of the following?
   1. Antigens
   2. Memory cells
   3. Complement
   4. Natural killer cells

3. Which of the following immunoglobulins is first produced during an acute infection?
   1. IgG
   2. IgM
   3. IgE
   4. IgD

4. Which of the following is the function of macrophages and neutrophils?
   1. Phagocytosis
   2. Antibody production
   3. Complement fixation
   4. Suppression of autoimmunity

5. The activation of B cells in humoral immunity is assisted by which of the following?
   1. Cytotoxic T cells
   2. Helper T cells
   3. Suppressor T cells
   4. Neutrophils

6. Autoimmunity is defined as a phenomenon involving which of the following?
   1. Production of endotoxins that destroy B lymphocytes.
   2. Inability to differentiate self from nonself.
   3. Overproduction of reagin antibody.
   4. Depression of the immune response.

REVIEW QUESTIONS—TEST PREPARATION

Choose the best answer unless directed otherwise.

7. Which of the following is used to determine the presence of inflammation? **Select all that apply.**
   1. IgM assay
   2. CD4+ count
   3. Western blot
   4. C-reactive protein (CRP)
   5. Erythrocyte sedimentation rate (ESR)

8. A mother brings her children into the clinic, and the children are diagnosed with chickenpox. The mother had chickenpox as a child. Which of the following statements should the nurse include in the patient teaching?
   1. "Because you have an active natural immunity to chickenpox, you can take care of the children at home."
   2. "You will need to wear a mask while caring for the children to prevent contamination."
   3. "You will need to get a booster chickenpox vaccination to ensure that you don't get reinfected."
   4. "Because you've had chickenpox before and your children are now ill, you should monitor yourself for signs or symptoms of shingles for the next 2 weeks."

9. Which of the following may stimulate antibody production? **Select all that apply.**
   1. Cold virus
   2. Plant pollen
   3. Transplanted organ
   4. Bacterial toxins
   5. Measles vaccine

10. The nurse is caring for a patient undergoing a biopsy. Which action is appropriate for the nurse to take?
    1. Ask whether the patient has an iodine allergy.
    2. Ensure that informed consent is obtained before the procedure.
    3. Ask the patient about environmental allergies and the type of reaction that occurs.
    4. Check eosinophil level on the laboratory report.

11. While working with patients in an autoimmune disease clinic, the nurse recognizes that which of the following individuals is most likely to develop systemic lupus erythematosus?
    1. A 38-year-old African American male who works in the construction industry
    2. A 55-year-old white female who works as a medical secretary
    3. A 19-year-old Asian female who is attending college
    4. A 34-year-old Native American male who works as a lawyer

VOCABULARY

Match the term with its definition.

1. _____ An anaphylactic-type reaction

2. _____ The type of antibodies that attach to mast cells

3. _____ Elimination of the offending environmental stimuli

4. _____ Very dry, pruritic, edematous skin

5. _____ Sudden, severe reaction characterized by smooth muscle spasms and capillary permeability changes

6. _____ Urticaria

7. _____ A form of lupus that affects only the skin

8. _____ Types of drugs used to prevent transplant rejection

9. _____ Painless subcutaneous and dermal erythremic eruptions with diffuse edema

10. _____ Requires lifelong vitamin B_{12}

11. _____ Red blood cell (RBC) fragments seen with microscope

12. _____ Infant may be asymptomatic until 6 months old

13. _____ Antimalarial and immunosuppressant drugs may be used in treatment

14. _____ Causes may include heat, cold, pressure, and stress

15. _____ Patient education includes a diet low in iodine and high in bulk, protein, and carbohydrates

16. _____ Patient education includes frequent movement and the use of a hard mattress and no pillow when sleeping

1. Urticaria
2. Angioedema
3. Anaphylaxis
4. Pernicious anemia
5. Hashimoto's thyroiditis
6. Idiopathic autoimmune hemolytic anemia
7. Hypogammaglobulinemia
8. Allergic rhinitis
9. Hives
10. Type I hypersensitivity reaction
11. Immunoglobulin (Ig)E
12. Ankylosing spondylitis
13. Atopic dermatitis
14. Immunosuppressive
15. Systemic lupus erythematosus
16. Discoid lupus erythematosus

IMMUNE DISORDERS

Fill in the blank.

1. The way hypersensitivity reactions are classified include _____, _____, _____, and _____.
2. When allergic rhinitis occurs seasonally, it is called _____.
3. Complications of allergic rhinitis are _____, _____, _____, and _____.
4. _____ is a complication of atopic dermatitis.
5. The first drug of choice for anaphylaxis is _____.
6. Urticaria is commonly called _____.
7. Angioedema differs from urticaria in that angioedema _____, _____, and _____.
8. The _____ is used to diagnose a hemolytic transfusion reaction.
9. _____ and _____ are two complications that can occur with a hemolytic transfusion reaction.
10. Today, serum sickness tends to occur when _____ and _____ are administered to patients.
11. _____ and _____ are two food additives that can trigger an anaphylactic reaction.
12. _____ is the most common cause of contact dermatitis.
13. Patients with pernicious anemia are unable to absorb _____.
14. _____ is a process whereby abnormal RBCs are removed and replaced with normal RBCs.
15. Ankylosing spondylitis is a chronic progressive inflammatory disease of the _____, _____, and _____ joints.

IMMUNE WORD SEARCH

Figure out what words the clues represent. Then find the words in the grid. Words can go horizontally, vertically, and diagonally in all eight directions.

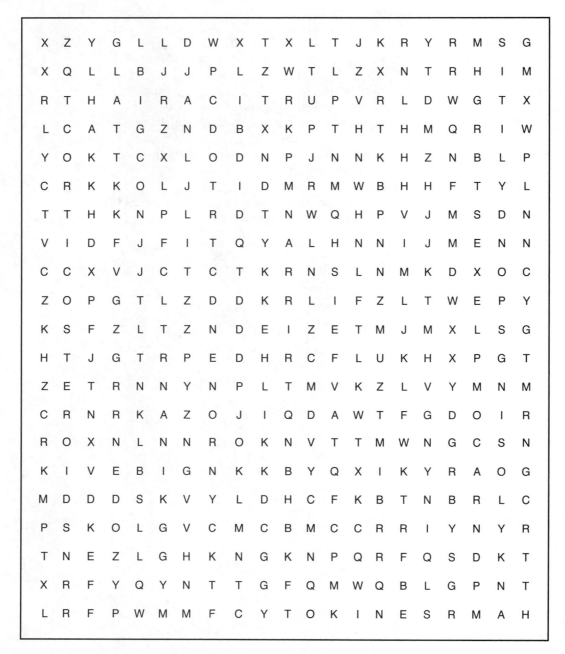

```
X Z Y G L L D W X T X L T J K R Y R M S G
X Q L L B J J P L Z W T L Z X N T R H I M
R T H A I R A C I T R U P V R L D W G T X
L C A T G Z N D B X K P T H T H M Q R I W
Y O K T C X L O D N P J N N K H Z N B L P
C R K K O L J T I D M R M W B H H F T Y L
T T H K N P L R D T N W Q H P V J M S D N
V I D F J F I T Q Y A L H N N I J M E N N
C C X V J C T C T K R N S L N M K D X O C
Z O P G T L Z D D K R L I F Z L T W E P Y
K S F Z L T Z N D E I Z E T M J M X L S G
H T J G T R P E D H R C F L U K H X P G T
Z E T R N N Y N P L T M V K Z L V Y M N M
C R N R K A Z O J I Q D A W T F G D O I R
R O X N L N N R O K N V T T M W N G C S N
K I V E B I G N K K B Y Q X I K Y R A O G
M D D D S K V Y L D H C F K B T N B R L C
P S K O L G V C M C B M C C R R I Y N Y R
T N E Z L G H K N G K N P Q R F Q S D K T
X R F Y Q Y N T T G F Q M W Q B L G P N T
L R F P W M M F C Y T O K I N E S R M A H
```

CLUES:
- When antigens clump.
- A nursing intervention for this disorder is a very firm mattress and no pillows when sleeping.
- A type I hypersensitivity that eventually leads to a thickening of the dermis with less sweat production in these areas.
- These are formed in type III hypersensitivity reactions, which then occlude blood vessels.
- These medications that are frequently used with immune system disorders should never be suddenly discontinued.
- Agents of the immune system that act to modify and enhance the immune and inflammatory responses.
- Type IV hypersensitivity reactions tend to be this—not immediate.
- These particular lymphocytes elevate in an allergic reaction as seen with type I hypersensitivities.
- The main complication for a patient with hypogammaglobulinemia.

IMMUNE PUZZLE

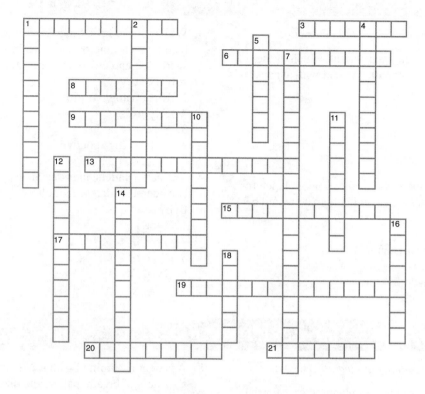

Across

1. A type of anemia that will develop in patients with autoimmune gastritis.
3. The number of minutes that a nurse should stay with a patient at the beginning of a blood transfusion.
6. This is a very serious type I hypersensitivity reaction.
8. An antibody-mediated response produced by B lymphocytes.
9. These phagocytic leukocytes are stationary.
13. Hashimoto's thyroiditis begins with this.
15. These are a complication of repeated episodes of allergic rhinitis.
17. Similar to urticaria although tends to be less pruritic, lasts longer, and involves deeper tissue.
19. The substance that is required in order for vitamin B_{12} to be absorbed in the small intestine.
20. This facial rash will occur in about 60% to 80% of systemic lupus erythematosus (SLE) patients.
21. This form of lupus erythematosus affects only the skin.

Down

1. Nowadays serum sickness tends to occur after administration of sulfonamides and these drugs.
2. A respiratory assessment finding that is considered an emergency in a patient with angioedema.
4. A drug of choice during an anaphylactic reaction.
5. This can overwhelmingly affect the activities of daily living (ADLs) of a patient with SLE.
7. This disorder is due to defective functioning B cells.
10. One group of joints that is affected in ankylosing spondylitis.
11. IgE antibodies attach to these cells in a type I hypersensitivity reaction.
12. Currently a significant type of contact dermatitis.
14. Ankylosing spondylitis is attributed to this.
16. A foreign protein or cell capable of causing an immune response.
18. An SLE flare trigger.

WORDS FOR IMMUNE PUZZLE

Allergen
Anaphylaxis
Angioedema
Autoimmunity
Butterfly
Discoid
Epinephrine
Fatigue

Fifteen
Humoral
Hypogammaglobulinemia
Hypothyroidism
Intrinsic factor
Latex allergy
Mast cells
Monocytes

Nasal polyps
Obstruction
Penicillins
Pernicious
Sacroiliac
Steroids
Stress

REVIEW QUESTIONS—CONTENT REVIEW

Choose the best answer unless directed otherwise.

1. As the nurse collects data on a patient, which of the following is a symptom that the patient with anaphylaxis may be experiencing?
   1. Dermatitis
   2. Delirium
   3. Sinusitis
   4. Wheezing

2. Which of the following is the medication of choice for anaphylaxis that the nurse should anticipate would be ordered?
   1. Epinephrine
   2. Theophylline (Theo-Dur)
   3. Digoxin (Lanoxin)
   4. Furosemide (Lasix)

3. Which of the following is a disease process characterized by a chronic progressive inflammation of the sacroiliac and costovertebral joints and adjacent soft tissue?
   1. Rheumatoid arthritis
   2. Kyphosis
   3. Scoliosis
   4. Ankylosing spondylitis

4. The nurse understands that an anaphylactic reaction is considered which of the following types of hypersensitivity reactions?
   1. Type I
   2. Type II
   3. Type III
   4. Type IV

REVIEW QUESTIONS—TEST PREPARATION

Choose the best answer unless directed otherwise.

5. A patient has allergic rhinitis. In planning care for the patient, the nurse understands that if the patient does not adhere to the treatment regimen, the patient is at risk for developing which of the following?
   1. Sinusitis
   2. Anaphylaxis
   3. Lymphadenopathy
   4. Angioedema

6. A patient reports on admission being "very sick" after taking erythromycin in the past. The patient is to receive erythromycin now. Which of the following actions should the nurse take regarding the antibiotic?
   1. Give the antibiotic.
   2. Give half of the dose.
   3. Do not give the antibiotic.
   4. Discontinue the antibiotic.

7. A patient is being given penicillin via intravenous (IV) infusion and develops an anaphylactic reaction. Which of the following should be the nurse's first action?
   1. Call the doctor.
   2. Call for help.
   3. Maintain the antibiotic.
   4. Turn off the antibiotic.

8. A patient is admitted with a 2-month history of fatigue, shortness of breath, pallor, and dizziness. The patient is diagnosed with idiopathic autoimmune hemolytic anemia. On reviewing the laboratory results, the nurse notes which of the following that confirms this diagnosis?
   1. RBC fragments
   2. Macrocytic, normochromic RBCs
   3. Microcytic, hypochromic RBCs
   4. Hemoglobin molecules

9. A patient had a portion of stomach removed and must take vitamin B_{12}. Which of the following statements should be included in the patient teaching?
   1. "You will develop iron-deficiency anemia if you fail to take vitamin B_{12}."
   2. "Pernicious anemia is a complication of this surgery, so you must take vitamin B_{12}."
   3. "Most patients who do not take vitamin B_{12} develop sickle cell anemia."
   4. "Taking vitamin B_{12} is important if you want to prevent acquired hemolytic anemia."

10. A patient is diagnosed with Hashimoto's thyroiditis and asks what causes it. The nurse would respond that the destruction of the thyroid in this condition is due to which of the following?
    1. Antigen-antibody complexes
    2. Autoantibodies
    3. Viral infection
    4. Bacterial infection

11. A patient who was walking in the woods disturbed a beehive, was stung, and was taken to the emergency department immediately due to allergies to bee stings. Which of the following symptoms would the nurse expect to see upon admission of this patient? **Select all that apply.**
    1. Pallor around the sting bites
    2. Numbness and tingling in the extremities
    3. Respiratory stridor
    4. Retinal hemorrhage
    5. Tachycardia
    6. Dyspnea

12. A patient has a long-standing history of allergies to pollen. Which of the following actions indicates that further teaching is necessary?
    1. The patient stays indoors on dry, windy days.
    2. The patient drives the car with the windows open.
    3. The patient avoids walking outside in the spring.
    4. The patient works in the garden on sunny days.

13. The nurse would evaluate that the patient understands what triggers allergic rhinitis by which of the following patient responses?
    1. "Injected medications"
    2. "Topical creams and ointments"
    3. "Ingested food and medications"
    4. "Airborne pollens and molds"

14. In caring for a patient with angioedema, the nurse understands that angioedema differs from urticaria in that angioedema is characterized by which of the following?
    1. Angioedema is more pruritic.
    2. Angioedema has a deeper and more widespread edema.
    3. Angioedema has small, fluid-filled vesicles that crust.
    4. Angioedema lasts a shorter time.

15. Which of the following is a common nursing diagnosis that the nurse will include in the plan of care for a patient with SLE?
    1. Fatigue
    2. Impaired Mobility
    3. Impaired Swallowing
    4. Impaired Tissue Perfusion

20 Nursing Care of Patients With HIV Disease and AIDS

VOCABULARY

Fill in the blank.

1. _____ is the final phase of a chronic, progressive immune function disorder caused by the human immunodeficiency virus (HIV).

2. The _____ cell is an important part of the human immune system and helps defend the body against very primitive invaders such as fungi, yeast, and other viruses.

3. _____ is a diagnostic test done to measure resistance to currently available antiviral treatments.

4. _____ are a primary complication of HIV infection and occur because of an impaired immune system.

5. _____ occurs in some patients with the acquired immune deficiency syndrome (AIDS) and is characterized by the occurrence of an involuntary baseline body weight loss of more than 10% and weakness or fever for more than 30 days or chronic diarrhea of two loose stools daily for more than 30 days.

6. _____ measures the amount of HIV RNA in plasma and is extremely important for determining prognosis and monitoring the response to antiretroviral therapy.

DIAGNOSTIC TESTS

Describe the procedure for each of the following diagnostic tests.

1. Enzyme-linked immunosorbent assay (ELISA) test

_____

_____

_____

2. Viral load

_____

_____

_____

_____

3. CD4+ cell count

_____

_____

_____

_____

4. Genotyping

_____

_____

_____

_____

HIV

Fill in the blanks.

1. HIV is transmitted through _____, _____, _____, and _____.

2. HIV may stay latent for _____ years.

3. Fatigue, headache, fever, and generalized lymph-adenopathy may be seen during the _____ stage of HIV infection.

4. _____ are increasingly becoming infected with HIV.

HIV AND AIDS

Indicate whether the following are true or false, and correct false statements.

1. If a health care worker is stuck with a needle from a patient with AIDS, exposure to the virus may occur even if gloves were worn. _____

2. HIV is caused by AIDS. _____

3. Individuals who are not men who have sex with men or who are intravenous (IV) drug users probably do not need to worry about contracting HIV and developing AIDS. _____

4. If the nurse suctions a patient with a fresh tracheostomy who is diagnosed with HIV and blood-tinged sputum gets in the nurse's eyes, the nurse may contract the virus. _____

5. Once a person is infected with HIV, the diagnosis can be made using laboratory tests within 1 to 2 days. _____

6. A patient with AIDS should always be placed into isolation for the protection of health care workers. _____

CRITICAL THINKING

Answer the following questions.

1. Jack Swope, age 26, has been diagnosed as HIV-positive. He asks, "Do I have AIDS and am I going to die?" What should you say to him?

_____

_____

_____

2. When is the patient with HIV considered to have AIDS?

_____

_____

_____

3. Jack is started on a combination of trimethoprim and sulfamethoxazole (Bactrim, Septra). Why?

_____

_____

_____

4. Later, Jack is diagnosed with AIDS with a CD4+ count of 200.

(a) Jack is 6 feet tall and weighs 135 lb. He is malnourished. What are possible reasons? _____

_____

_____

(b) What can you do as a nurse to improve Jack's nutrition?

_____

_____

_____

5. Six months after being diagnosed with AIDS, Jack develops dementia. Why?

_____

_____

_____

6. How can a nurse contract HIV from a patient?

_____

_____

_____

7. How should the home health nurse teach family members of a patient with AIDS to clean the patient's home?

_____

_____

_____

REVIEW QUESTIONS—CONTENT REVIEW

Choose the best answer unless directed otherwise.

1. Which of the following best defines acquired immuno-deficiency syndrome (AIDS)?
   1. AIDS is a syndrome that always develops after infection with HIV virus.
   2. AIDS is the final phase of a chronic progressive immune disorder caused by HIV.
   3. AIDS is caused by HIV and characterized by CD4+ T lymphocytes greater than 14% of total lymphocytes.
   4. AIDS is an acute syndrome that is accompanied by specific clinical conditions.

2. For most HIV-infected patients being treated with antiviral medications, CBC, CD4+/C8+ T-lymphocyte count, and viral load testing are repeated at what intervals?
   1. Every month
   2. Every 3 months
   3. Every 6 months
   4. Every 12 months

REVIEW QUESTIONS—TEST PREPARATION

Choose the best answer unless directed otherwise.

3. In planning an educational session for a patient with HIV, the nurse would include which of the following as a method of transmission for HIV? **Select all that apply.**
   1. Saliva
   2. Tears
   3. Breast milk
   4. Semen
   5. Blood
   6. Sweat

4. A patient who is being tested for HIV asks what tests are used. The nurse would be correct in stating that the tests used to confirm HIV infection include which of the following?
   1. CD4+ cell count and thymus function
   2. B-cell and T-cell count
   3. ELISA and Western blot
   4. CD4+, viral load, and ELISA

5. The nurse is caring for a patient with HIV who has diarrhea. Which of the following would be most therapeutic to teach the patient to avoid in the diet to reduce diarrhea?
   1. Potassium-rich food
   2. Raw fruits and vegetables
   3. Liquid nutritional supplements
   4. Frozen products

6. The nurse is teaching a patient newly diagnosed with AIDS about complications of the disease. Which of the following is the most common opportunistic infection in AIDS?
   1. *Pneumocystis* pneumonia
   2. Candidiasis
   3. Toxoplasmosis
   4. *Mycoplasma* pneumonia

7. The nurse is taking vital signs of a pregnant woman during her first prenatal visit. The patient asks the nurse if she has to have an HIV test. Which of the following is the nurse's best response?
   1. "Yes, all pregnant women must have the test."
   2. "If you do not have multiple sex partners or inject drugs, it is not necessary."
   3. "Governmental guidelines require an HIV test for all pregnant woman."
   4. "After voluntary pretest counseling, you decide whether HIV testing should be done."

8. The nurse is caring for a patient with HIV. Which of the following foods would the nurse teach the patient is safe to eat to reduce the risk of infection?
   1. Raw fruits
   2. Cooked vegetables
   3. Raw vegetables
   4. Caesar dressing

9. When caring for a patient with AIDS, which of the following nursing actions would be most appropriate for infection control?
   1. Wear gloves at all times.
   2. Wear gloves for blood/body fluid contact.
   3. Wear gown and mask at all times.
   4. Wear a mask during patient contact times.

10. The nurse is asked if male circumcision has any relationship to HIV. Which of the following responses by the nurse is best?
    1. "Circumcision in male infants is strictly a religious preference."
    2. "Males who have been circumcised are more likely to acquire HIV with homosexual contact."
    3. "No research is available to indicate a relationship between HIV and circumcision."
    4. "There is evidence that males engaged in heterosexual activity are less likely to be infected with HIV if they've been circumcised."

unit FIVE

Understanding the Cardiovascular System

CHECKLIST FOR LEARNING SUCCESS

Review of Anatomy and Physiology and Aging Changes	Major Disorders	Nursing Assessment	Diagnostic Tests	Common Interventions
❑ Cardiovascular:	Cardiovascular:	❑ Medical history	❑ Electrocardiogram	❑ Exercise
❑ Structures	❑ Hypertension	❑ Medications	❑ Computerized tomography	❑ Smoking cessation
❑ Function	❑ Valvular	❑ Family history	❑ Cardiac magnetic resonance imaging	❑ Diet
❑ Aging effects	❑ Inflammatory	❑ Health promotion	❑ Exercise stress testing	❑ Lifestyle and cardiac care
	❑ Infectious	❑ Vital signs	❑ Echocardiogram	❑ Antiembolism devices
	❑ Occlusive	❑ Physical examination	❑ Tilt table test	❑ Cardioversion/defibrillation
	❑ Dysrhythmias		❑ Radioisotope imaging	❑ Pacemaker
	❑ Heart failure		❑ Cardiac enzymes	❑ Angioplasty
			❑ Cardiac troponin	❑ Valvuloplasty
			❑ Myoglobin	❑ Surgery
			❑ Homocysteine	❑ Cardiac rehabilitation
			❑ Lipids	
			❑ Angiography	
			❑ Cardiac catheterization	

21 Cardiovascular System Function, Assessment, and Therapeutic Measures

STRUCTURES OF THE CARDIOVASCULAR SYSTEM

Label the following structures.

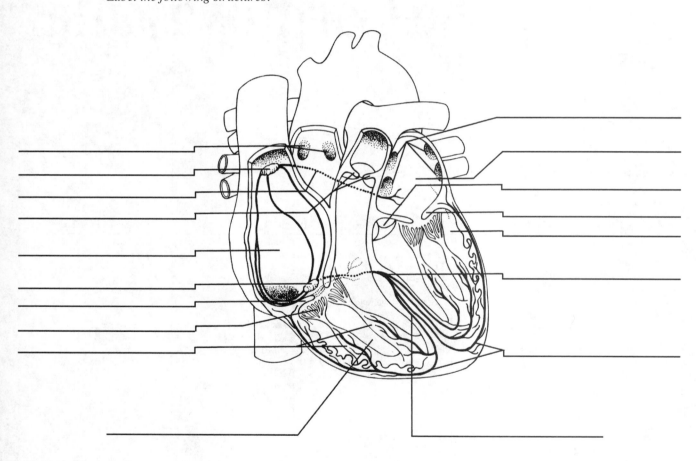

CARDIAC BLOOD FLOW

Number the following in proper sequence with respect to the flow of blood through the heart and to and from the lungs and body. Begin with the caval veins.

1. _____ Superior and inferior caval veins
2. _____ Left ventricle
3. _____ Right atrium
4. _____ Right ventricle
5. _____ Body

6. _____ Lungs
7. _____ Pulmonary artery
8. _____ Pulmonary veins
9. _____ Aorta
10. _____ Left atrium

11. _____ Mitral valve
12. _____ Aortic valve
13. _____ Tricuspid valve
14. _____ Pulmonic valve

AGING AND THE CARDIOVASCULAR SYSTEM

Find the 11 errors and insert the correct information.

It is believed that the "aging" of blood vessels, especially arteries, begins in adulthood. Average resting blood pressure tends to decrease with age and may contribute to stroke or right-sided heart failure. The thicker walled veins, especially those of the legs, may also weaken and stretch, making their valves incompetent.

    With age, the heart lining becomes less efficient, and there is an increase in both maximum cardiac output and heart rate. The health of the myocardium depends on the lungs' blood supply. Hypertension causes the right ventricle to work harder, so it may atrophy. The heart valves may become thinner from fibrosis, leading to heart murmurs. Dysrhythmias become more common in older adults as the cells of the conduction pathway become more efficient.

CARDIOVASCULAR SYSTEM

Fill in the blanks.

1. The function of the _____ is to carry oxygen and nutrients to the tissues and remove waste products.
2. The _____ function is to pump blood.
3. The peripheral _____ is composed of arteries, veins, _____ and lymph vessels.
4. With aging, the walls of blood vessels _____.
5. The heart sound _____ occurs at the beginning of systole when the atrioventricular valves close, and the sound *dupp* occurs at the start of _____ when the semilunar valves close.
6. Palpation of pulse quality is recorded as _____ 0; weak, thready 1+; _____ 2+; bounding 3+.
7. Tests to assess _____ function may include x-ray examination, electrocardiogram (ECG), stress test, echocardiogram, thallium scan, dipyridamole thallium scan, multiple gated acquisition (MUGA), serum troponin I, creatine kinase, (CK-MB), myoglobin, cardiac _____, and angiography.
8. The six Ps characterize _____ vascular disease: _____, _____ pulselessness, pallor, paresthesia, and paralysis.

9. Tests to assess peripheral _____ disease are plethysmography, Doppler ultrasound, pressure measurement, stress testing, _____, and arteriography.

ACUTE CARDIOVASCULAR NURSING ASSESSMENT

Identify a word that is obtained during a history that matches the given assessment statement.

1. _____ Assessed before medication administration, test dyes
2. _____ Modifiable risk factor for cardiovascular disorders that is a habit
3. _____ Location: chest, calf; radiation: arms, jaw neck
4. _____ Sign resulting from right-sided heart failure
5. _____ Lung sounds with left-sided heart failure
6. _____ Symptom of dysrhythmias
7. _____ Effect of decreased cardiac output
8. _____ Classic symptom of acute heart failure (pulmonary edema)

CRITICAL THINKING

Make a concept map for a patient who is to undergo a cardiac catheterization. A concept map helps you visualize the patient's needs. Think of possible categories of needs of this patient and then complete activities and needs under each category. Some categories have been given to get you started, but you may think of others to include. You can get even more detailed and create subcategories for each activity or need. A concept map has no defined ending point. See Davis*Plus*, an F.A. Davis Internet site that provides nursing resources, for a program that has been provided to help you create concept maps.

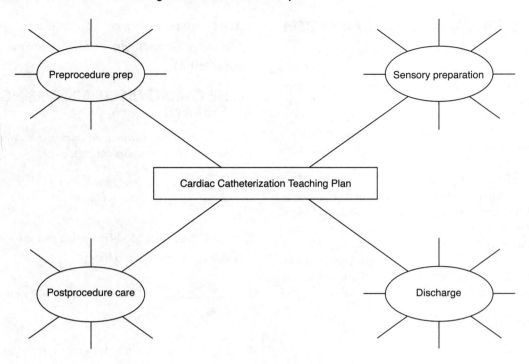

REVIEW QUESTIONS—CONTENT REVIEW

Choose the best answer unless directed otherwise.

1. Each normal heartbeat is initiated by which of the following?
   1. Sinoatrial node in the wall of the right atrium
   2. Bundle of His in the interventricular septum
   3. Cardiac center in the medulla
   4. Sympathetic nerves from the spinal cord

2. During one cardiac cycle, which of the following occurs?
   1. Ventricles contract first, followed by the atria
   2. Atria contract first, followed by the ventricles
   3. Atria and ventricles contract simultaneously
   4. Ventricles contract twice for every contraction of the atria

3. Which of the following detects changes in blood pressure?
   1. Pressoreceptors in the medulla
   2. Blood vessels in the medulla
   3. Pressoreceptors in the carotid and aortic sinuses
   4. Coronary vessels in the myocardium

4. Epinephrine increases blood pressure because it does which of the following?
   1. Increases water resorption by the kidneys
   2. Causes vasodilation in the skin and viscera
   3. Decreases heart rate and force of contraction
   4. Increases heart rate and force of cardiac contraction

5. When blood pressure decreases, the kidneys help raise it by secreting which of the following?
   1. Renin
   2. Epinephrine
   3. Aldosterone
   4. Erythropoietin

6. Which of the following prevents the backflow of blood in veins?
   1. Precapillary sphincters
   2. Middle layer
   3. Smooth muscle layer
   4. Valves

7. The mitral and tricuspid valves prevent backflow of blood from which of the following?
   1. Ventricles to atria when the ventricles contract
   2. Atria to ventricles when the ventricles relax
   3. Ventricles to atria when the atria contract
   4. Atria to ventricles when the atria contract

8. Which of the following describes the purpose of the endocardium of the heart?
   1. Covers the heart muscle and prevents friction.
   2. Supports the coronary blood vessels.
   3. Lines the chambers of the heart and prevents abnormal clotting.
   4. Prevents backflow of blood from atria to ventricles.

9. Which of the following is the function of the coronary arteries?
   1. Prevent abnormal clotting within the heart.
   2. Bring oxygenated blood to the myocardium.
   3. Carry deoxygenated blood to the lungs.
   4. Carry oxygenated blood to the lungs.

10. Where in the nervous system is the cardiac center found?
    1. Cerebrum
    2. Hypothalamus
    3. Spinal cord
    4. Medulla

11. Angiotensin II increases which of the following?
    1. Vasodilation and antidiuretic hormone (ADH) secretion
    2. Vasoconstriction and aldosterone secretion
    3. Heart rate and vasodilation
    4. Heart rate and ADH secretion

12. The increase of resting blood pressure with age may contribute to which of the following?
    1. Dysrhythmias
    2. Thrombus formation
    3. Left-sided heart failure
    4. Peripheral edema

REVIEW QUESTIONS—TEST PREPARATION

Choose the best answer unless directed otherwise.

13. A patient had a bilateral mastectomy 2 days ago, so the nurse obtains blood pressure readings from the patient's legs. The patient's baseline blood pressure in the arm was 112/78 mm Hg. Which of the following readings, when compared with baseline blood pressure, does the nurse expect when taking the blood pressure in the leg?
    1. 122/84 mm Hg
    2. 102/68 mm Hg
    3. 132/78 mm Hg
    4. 96/58 mm Hg

14. The nurse obtains a lower blood pressure reading on a patient's left arm than the right arm. As a result, which of the following extremities should the nurse use for ongoing blood pressure measurement?
    1. Left arm
    2. Right arm
    3. Right leg
    4. Either arm

15. The nurse is checking a patient's blood pressure for orthostatic hypotension. The patient's BP lying down was 142/88 mm Hg and 136/80 mm Hg when standing. The patient asks the nurse why there is such a difference. Which of the following is the best response by the nurse?
    1. "Your blood pressure should go up about 15 mm Hg, so we'll need to have you move very slowly to avoid a fall."
    2. "Blood pressure usually compensates for a change in position by going down by about 15 mm Hg, so this is normal."
    3. "It is safe for the blood pressure to drop by as much as 25 mm Hg, so you don't need to worry."
    4. "Your blood pressure is still in a normal range so there is no real concern."

16. A patient's pulse is 78 beats per minute (beats/min) and blood pressure (BP) = 122/76 mm Hg while lying down. While the nurse checks the patient's blood pressure for orthostatic hypotension, the patient's heart rate increases to 92 beats/min, and the BP = 116/68 mm Hg. Which of the following actions should the nurse take?
    1. Return the patient to a lying position immediately.
    2. Ask if the patient is experiencing chest pain.
    3. Note that normal compensation occurred.
    4. Chart that the patient has orthostatic hypotension.

17. The nurse is inspecting a patient's legs for data collection and notes that there is bilateral decreased hair distribution, thick, brittle nails, and shiny, taut, dry skin. The nurse understands that this can indicate which of the following?
    1. Increased arterial blood flow
    2. Decreased arterial blood flow
    3. Increased venous blood flow
    4. Decreased venous blood flow

18. The nurse is explaining to a patient that for a thallium stress test dipyridamole (Persantine), a coronary vasodilator, will be given. Which of the following would the nurse include in the teaching regarding the reason this medication is being given?
    1. To decrease blood flow to cardiac cells
    2. To increase blood flow as exercise would
    3. To prevent a clot from forming during the test
    4. To reduce systemic vascular resistance

19. Which of the following data would be most important for the nurse to collect immediately for a patient who is reporting fatigue and dizziness? **Select all that apply.**
    1. Presence of pain
    2. Weight
    3. Vital signs
    4. Electrocardiogram tracing
    5. White blood cell count
    6. Palpitations

22 Nursing Care of Patients With Hypertension

VOCABULARY

Match the word with its definition.

1. _____ Atherosclerosis
2. _____ Peripheral vascular resistance
3. _____ Normotensive
4. _____ Isolated systolic hypertension
5. _____ Hypertension
6. _____ Diastolic blood pressure
7. _____ Cardiac output
8. _____ Systolic blood pressure
9. _____ Secondary hypertension
10. _____ Primary hypertension
11. _____ Plaque

1. Most common form of arteriosclerosis, in which fats are deposited on arterial walls
2. Amount of blood the heart pumps out each minute
3. Amount of pressure exerted on the wall of the arteries when the ventricles are at rest; the bottom number in a blood pressure reading
4. Abnormally elevated blood pressure
5. Systolic pressure is 140 mm Hg or more, but the diastolic pressure is less than 90 mm Hg
6. Normal blood pressure
7. Opposition to blood flow through the vessels
8. Deposit of fatty material in the artery
9. Abnormally elevated blood pressure, the cause of which is unknown; also called essential hypertension
10. High blood pressure that is a symptom of a specific cause, such as a kidney abnormality
11. Maximal pressure exerted on the arteries during contraction of the left ventricle of the heart; top number of a blood pressure reading

DIURETICS

Select the number that identifies the type of each diuretic.

1. _____ Spironolactone (Aldactone)
2. _____ Bumetanide (Bumex)
3. _____ Chlorothiazide (Diuril)
4. _____ Triamterene (Dyrenium)
5. _____ Furosemide (Lasix)
6. _____ Amiloride (Midamor)
7. _____ Metolazone (Zaroxolyn)
8. _____ Hydrochlorothiazide
9. _____ Torsemide (Demadex)

1. Thiazide or thiazide-like
2. Loop
3. Potassium sparing

HYPERTENSION RISK FACTORS

Indicate whether the statement is true or false.

1. _____ Increased stress can cause hypertension.
2. _____ There is a link between a high-fat diet, obesity, and hypertension.
3. _____ High calcium, potassium, and magnesium levels are important risk factors for the development of hypertension.
4. _____ People who are not active on a regular basis are at an increased risk of developing hypertension.
5. _____ A diet high in salt is also high in vitamins and minerals.
6. _____ Inadequate sleep of less than 5 hours is a risk factor for hypertension.
7. _____ Classical music for 30 minutes daily can reduce blood pressure.

STAGES OF HYPERTENSION AND RECOMMENDATIONS FOR FOLLOW-UP

Indicate whether the statement is true or false and correct the false statements.

1. _____ The recommended follow-up for a systolic blood pressure of 120 to 139 mm Hg is 2 years.
2. _____ The recommended follow-up for a systolic blood pressure of less than 120 mm Hg is 2 years.
3. _____ The recommended follow-up for a systolic blood pressure more than 180 mm Hg is right now.
4. _____ The recommended follow-up for a systolic blood pressure of 160 to 179 mm Hg is 2 months.
5. _____ The recommended follow-up for a systolic blood pressure of 140 to 159 mm Hg is 2 months.
6. _____ The recommended follow-up for a diastolic blood pressure of 90 to 99 mm Hg is 1 month.
7. _____ The recommended follow-up for a diastolic blood pressure of more than 110 mm Hg is right now.
8. _____ The recommended follow-up for a diastolic blood pressure of 100 to 109 mm Hg is 2 months.
9. _____ The recommended follow-up for a diastolic blood pressure less than 80 mm Hg is 2 years.
10. _____ The recommended follow-up for a diastolic blood pressure of 80 to 89 mm Hg is 1 year.

CRITICAL THINKING

Read the following case study and answer the questions.

Mrs. Laura Martin, age 42, is seen in the hypertension clinic for a follow-up visit for hypertension. Her blood pressure is 160/92 mm Hg, and she is diagnosed with hypertension. The health care provider encourages continued lifestyle modification and prescribes hydrochlorothiazide.

1. Why is hydrochlorothiazide prescribed? _____
   _____
   _____

2. What additional information should the nurse collect to develop a teaching plan for lifestyle modifications and the medication? _____
   _____
   _____

3. Develop a teaching plan for Mrs. Martin's needs based on the data collected. _____
   _____
   _____

4. What interventions will help Mrs. Martin reach her goal for controlling her hypertension? _____

_____

_____

5. How will you know when Mrs. Martin has reached her goals? _____

_____

_____

REVIEW QUESTIONS—CONTENT REVIEW

Choose the best answer unless directed otherwise.

1. If the systolic blood pressure is elevated and the diastolic blood pressure is normal, the nurse recognizes that a patient is most likely to have which type of hypertension?
   1. Primary
   2. Secondary
   3. Isolated systolic

2. The nurse explains to a patient with blood pressure readings of 164/102 mm Hg and 176/100 mm Hg on two separate occasions that this type of hypertension is classified in which hypertension category?
   1. Prehypertension
   2. Stage 1
   3. Stage 2

3. The nurse would explain to the patient that the action of enalapril maleate (Vasotec) is which of the following?
   1. It decreases levels of angiotensin II.
   2. It adjusts the extracellular volume.
   3. It dilates the arterioles and veins.
   4. It decreases cardiac output.

4. The nurse understands that which of the following best describes the action of propranolol (Inderal) to teach the patient about the action of this medication?
   1. It increases heart rate.
   2. It decreases cardiac output.
   3. It decreases fluid volume.
   4. It increases cardiac contractility.

REVIEW QUESTIONS—TEST PREPARATION

Choose the best answer unless directed otherwise.

5. The nurse is developing a teaching plan for a patient. Which of the following is a modifiable risk factor for the development of hypertension? **Select all that apply.**
   1. Race
   2. High cholesterol
   3. Cigarette smoking
   4. Sedentary lifestyle
   5. Less than 5 hours of sleep

6. The patient asks the nurse, "How is hypertension defined?" Which of the following is the best response by the nurse?
   1. "It is measured as the heart pumps blood into the arteries."
   2. "It is blood pressure above 140/90 mm Hg on two separate occasions."
   3. "It is regulated by stress, activity, and emotions."
   4. "It is determined by peripheral vascular resistance."

7. Which of the following should the nurse include when counseling a patient about smoking and its effect on blood pressure?
   1. Smoking is associated with stages 1 and 2 hypertension.
   2. Smoking does not affect blood pressure regulation.
   3. Smoking vasodilates the peripheral blood vessels.
   4. Smoking causes sustained blood pressure elevations.

8. A patient calls the hypertension clinic to report frequent headaches with a newly prescribed medication. The nurse anticipates that this is a normal side effect if the patient is taking which of the following medications?
   1. Furosemide (Lasix)
   2. Atenolol (Tenormin)
   3. Clonidine (Catapres)
   4. Adalat (Procardia)

9. A patient has been prescribed bumetanide (Bumex) every morning for control of hypertension. Which of the following statements indicates correct knowledge of the treatment regimen?
   1. "I can travel to Florida and sunbathe all day."
   2. "Now I can eat whatever I want, whenever I want."
   3. "I'll take my medication in the morning, every morning."
   4. "I won't need medication once my pressure goes down."

10. Which common side effect of metolazone (Zaroxolyn) should the nurse instruct a patient to report to the health care provider?
    1. Numb hands
    2. Muscle weakness
    3. Gastrointestinal distress
    4. Nightmares

11. The nurse understands that which of the following is a side effect most likely to be reported by patients receiving enalapril maleate (Vasotec)?
    1. Acne
    2. Diarrhea
    3. Cough
    4. Heartburn

12. What instruction should the nurse give to the patient taking propranolol (Inderal) for hypertension?
    1. Have potassium level checked.
    2. Report any changes in appetite.
    3. Do not stop medication abruptly.
    4. Resume usual daily activities.

13. Which of the following nursing diagnoses is the focus of care for a patient with hypertension?
    1. Activity Intolerance
    2. Ineffective Airway Clearance
    3. Impaired Physical Mobility
    4. Deficient Knowledge

14. Which of the following statements, if made by a patient with hypertension, indicates to the nurse a need for more teaching?
    1. "High blood pressure may affect the kidneys and eyes."
    2. "Most people with hypertension watch their diet."
    3. "Medication will no longer be needed when I feel better."
    4. "Many people do not know when their blood pressure is high."

15. The nurse is developing a patient teaching plan. The teaching plan should include which of the following lifestyle modifications to help control hypertension?
    1. Regular aerobic exercise
    2. Low-tar cigarettes
    3. Three alcoholic beverages per day
    4. Daily multivitamin supplements

23

Nursing Care of Patients With Valvular, Inflammatory, and Infectious Cardiac or Venous Disorders

VOCABULARY

Fill in the blank with the word that is formed by the word building.

1. _____ annulus—ring + plasty—formed
2. _____ commissura—joining together + tome—incision
3. _____ in—not + sufficiens—sufficient
4. _____ re—again + gurgitare—to flood
5. _____ stenos—narrow
6. _____ valvula—leaf of a folding door + plasty—formed
7. _____ choreia—dance
8. _____ peri—around + kardia—heart + itis—inflammation
9. _____ myo—muscle + kardia—heart + itis—inflammation
10. _____ petecchia—skin spot
11. _____ peri—around + kardia—heart + kentesis—puncture
12. _____ kardia—heart + tamponade—plug
13. _____ kardia—heart + myo—muscle + pathy—disease
14. _____ kardia—heart + mega—large
15. _____ my—muscle + ectomy—cutting out
16. _____ thromb—lump (clot) + phleb—vein + itis—inflammation

MITRAL VALVE PROLAPSE

Find the eight errors and insert the correct information.

During ventricular diastole, when pressures in the left ventricle rise, the leaflets of the mitral valve normally remain open. In mitral valve prolapse (MVP), however, the leaflets bulge backward into the left ventricle during systole. Often there are functional problems seen with MVP. However, if the leaflets do not fit together, mitral stenosis can occur with varying degrees of severity.

MVP tends to be hereditary, and the cause is known. Infections that damage the mitral valve may be a contributing factor. It is the most common form of valvular heart disease and typically occurs in men aged 20 to 55. Most patients with MVP have symptoms. Symptoms that may occur include chest pain, dysrhythmias, palpitations, dizziness, and syncope. No treatment is needed unless symptoms are present. Stimulants and caffeine should be avoided to prevent symptoms.

VALVULAR DISORDERS

Indicate whether the statement is true or false and correct false statements.

1. _____ Stenosis is widening of the opening of a heart valve.

2. _____ Stenosis inhibits the forward flow of blood.

3. _____ Regurgitation, or insufficiency, is failure of the valve to close completely.

4. _____ Regurgitation inhibits backflow of blood.

5. _____ Rheumatic heart disease and congenital defects are primary causes of valvular disease.

6. _____ The primary valves affected by disease are the tricuspid and pulmonic valves.

7. _____ Compensatory mechanisms in valvular disease are dilation to handle the increased blood volume and hypertrophy to increase the strength of contractions.

8. _____ Symptoms of valvular disease often occur early and reflect decreased cardiac output and pulmonary congestion: fatigue, dyspnea, orthopnea, cough.

9. _____ In severe valvular disease, heart failure occurs, and symptoms reflect the backup of blood from the failing chamber.

10. _____ In acute valve disorders, symptoms of shock are seen.

11. _____ Valve disease diagnosis is made with electrocardiogram (ECG), chest x-ray examination, echocardiogram, and cardiac catheterization.

12. _____ Valvuloplasty uses a balloon to separate the valve leaflets.

13. _____ Commissurotomy narrows the valve opening.

14. _____ Annuloplasty surgically repairs the valve.

15. _____ Patient teaching for valvular disorders includes understanding the importance of prophylactic antibiotics before all invasive procedures.

CRITICAL THINKING—MRS. MURPHY

Read the case study and answer the questions.

Mrs. Murphy, age 72, has aortic stenosis and is scheduled for an aortic valve replacement. She reports fatigue and dyspnea with exertion.

1. What may be the cause of Mrs. Murphy's aortic stenosis?

_____

_____

_____

2. When obtaining Mrs. Murphy's medical history, what should the nurse ask that is relevant to the cause of aortic stenosis?

_____

_____

_____

3. How does the heart compensate for aortic stenosis?

_____

_____

_____

4. What should the nurse anticipate may occur in severe aortic stenosis?

_____

_____

_____

5. Why is angina a common symptom of aortic stenosis?

_____

_____

_____

6. Why does Mrs. Murphy's chest x-ray examination show an enlarged heart?

_____

_____

_____

7. Why is aortic stenosis treated with valvular replacement?

_____

_____

_____

INFLAMMATORY AND INFECTIOUS CARDIOVASCULAR DISORDERS

Match the word with its definition.

1. _____ Solid, liquid, gaseous masses of undissolved matter traveling with the current in a blood or lymphatic vessel.
2. _____ Gram-positive bacteria whose group A causes disease.
3. _____ Inflammation of the heart lining caused by microorganisms.
4. _____ Standardized test for reporting prothrombin to prevent variability in testing results and provide uniformity in monitoring therapeutic levels for coagulation.
5. _____ Severe damage to the heart from rheumatic fever.

1. Infective endocarditis
2. Emboli
3. International normalized ratio
4. Rheumatic heart disease
5. Beta-hemolytic streptococci

RHEUMATIC FEVER AND RHEUMATIC HEART DISEASE

Find the six errors and insert the correct information.

Rheumatic fever causes a streptococcal infection such as a sore throat. Rheumatic fever signs and symptoms include polyarthritis, subcutaneous nodules, cholera with rapid and controlled movements, carditis, fever, arthralgia, and pneumonia. A throat culture diagnoses rheumatic fever. The heart valves and their structures can be scarred and damaged. Rheumatic fever can be prevented by detecting and treating streptococcal infections promptly with aspirin.

DIAGNOSTIC TESTS FOR INFECTIVE ENDOCARDITIS

Match the test with its finding that is indicative of infective endocarditis.

Test

1. _____ White blood cell (WBC) count
2. _____ Blood cultures
3. _____ Electrocardiogram
4. _____ Chest x-ray examination
5. _____ Echocardiogram

Finding

1. Vegetations on heart valves
2. Dysrhythmias
3. Slight elevation
4. Heart failure
5. Identifies causative organism

THROMBOPHLEBITIS

Complete the rationale and evaluation of the nursing care plan for a patient with thrombophlebitis.

NURSING DIAGNOSIS
Acute Pain *related to inflammation of vein*

Interventions	Rationale	Evaluation
Assess pain using rating scale such as 0 to 10.		
Provide analgesics and nonsteroidal anti-inflammatory drugs (NSAIDs) as ordered.		
Apply warm, moist soaks.		
Maintain bedrest with leg elevation above heart level.		

NURSING DIAGNOSIS

Deficient Knowledge *related to lack of knowledge about disorder and treatment*

Interventions	Rationale	Evaluation
Explain condition, symptoms, and complications.		
Explain medications, therapies ordered, monthly lab test monitoring, and need for medical identification.		
Teach patient not to massage extremity.		

CRITICAL THINKING—MR. EVANS

Read the case study and answer the questions.

Mr. Evans, age 68, is admitted to the hospital for heart failure resulting from hypertrophic cardiomyopathy. He has dyspnea, fatigue, and angina. His lung sounds reveal crackles.

1. What is the pathophysiology of hypertrophic cardiomyopathy? _____

_____

_____

2. What occurs in hypertrophic cardiomyopathy to ventricular size and ventricular filling with blood? _____

_____

_____

3. What diagnostic test will show hypertrophic cardiomyopathy and left-sided heart failure? _____

_____

_____

4. Why is digoxin contraindicated for Mr. Evans?

_____

_____

_____

5. Why should Mr. Evans be taught to avoid (a) dehydration and (b) exertion? _____

_____

_____

6. Why is it important for the family to learn cardiopulmonary resuscitation (CPR)? _____

_____

_____

REVIEW QUESTIONS—CONTENT REVIEW

Choose the best answer unless directed otherwise.

1. Which of the following does the nurse understand occurs in aortic stenosis?
   1. Aortic valve does not close tightly.
   2. Emptying of blood from left ventricle is impaired.
   3. Blood backflows into the left atrium.
   4. Emptying of the left atrium is impaired.

2. The nurse understands that which of the following occurs in mitral regurgitation?
   1. Backflow of blood into the left atrium
   2. Backflow of blood into the right atrium
   3. Impaired emptying of the right ventricle
   4. Impaired emptying of the left ventricle

3. Which of the following compensatory mechanisms does the nurse understand occurs with ventricular valve disorders?
   1. Decreased atrial kick
   2. Atrial hypertrophy
   3. Ventricular hypertrophy
   4. Systolic hypertension

4. Which of the following does the nurse understand causes fatigue in patients with chronic aortic stenosis?
   1. Atrial fibrillation
   2. Left ventricular failure
   3. Decreased pulmonary blood flow
   4. Increased coronary artery blood flow

5. Which of the following diagnostic tests does the nurse understand measures the pressures in the cardiac chambers?
   1. Electrocardiogram
   2. Exercise stress test
   3. Echocardiogram
   4. Cardiac catheterization

6. Which of the following does the nurse understand usually precedes rheumatic fever?
   1. A viral infection
   2. A fungal infection
   3. A staphylococcal infection
   4. A beta-hemolytic streptococcal infection

7. Which of the following is the most common symptom of pericarditis?
   1. Dyspnea
   2. Intermittent claudication
   3. Chest pain
   4. Calf pain

REVIEW QUESTIONS—TEST PREPARATION

Choose the best answer unless directed otherwise.

8. Which of the following should the nurse include in the plan of care as a patient outcome for *Deficient Knowledge* related to mitral stenosis?
   1. Clear breath sounds, no edema or weight gain.
   2. Normal changes in vital signs with less fatigue during self-care.
   3. Verbalizes knowledge of disorder.
   4. States fear is reduced.

9. Which of the following medications does the nurse anticipate that the patient will be given to prevent complications associated with decreased cardiac output?
   Select all that apply.
   1. Furosemide (Lasix)
   2. Cephalexin (Keflex)
   3. Penicillin (Bicillin)
   4. Warfarin (Coumadin)
   5. rPA (Retavase)
   6. Potassium supplement

10. The nurse is caring for a patient, age 70, who has a nursing diagnosis of *Deficient Knowledge* related to furosemide administration. Which of the following interventions is essential to include when planning a teaching session?
    1. Determine patient's learning priorities.
    2. Tell patient what to learn first about furosemide.
    3. Assess patient's dietary intake of potassium.
    4. Give patient a written test at the end of the teaching session.

11. A patient, age 65, is being discharged after a mechanical valve replacement for aortic stenosis. Which of the following should be taught regarding warfarin (Coumadin) therapy?
    1. Wear medical identification.
    2. Increase intake of green leafy vegetables.
    3. Keep yearly blood test appointments.
    4. Use a straight razor when shaving.

12. The nurse is teaching a patient with heart failure how to avoid activity that results in Valsalva's maneuver. Which of the following statements by the patient indicates to the nurse that the teaching has been effective?
    1. "I will breathe normally when moving."
    2. "I will use a straw to drink oral fluids."
    3. "I will take fewer but deeper breaths."
    4. "I will clench my teeth when moving."

13. The nurse is planning care for a patient with chronic mitral regurgitation. Which of the following assessments would be the highest priority?
    1. Cardiac rhythm
    2. Heart tones
    3. Peripheral edema
    4. Lung sounds

14. A patient with a history of endocarditis is undergoing dental work and is recommended to take prophylactic antibiotics to prevent which of the following?
    1. Infective endocarditis
    2. Peritonitis
    3. Vegetative emboli
    4. Inflammation

15. A patient has a positive Homans' sign. Which of the following does the nurse understand explains why ambulation and performing the Homans' sign is now contraindicated?
    1. They can cause calf swelling.
    2. They can cause patient pain.
    3. They can cause emboli.
    4. They may cause a clot to form.

16. A patient develops a postoperative deep venous thrombosis and is started on intravenous (IV) heparin. Which of the following laboratory tests does the nurse monitor during heparin therapy?
    1. Plasma fibrinogen
    2. Prothrombin time (PT)
    3. Partial thromboplastin time (PTT)
    4. International normalized ratio (INR)

17. The nurse is caring for a patient on warfarin (Coumadin) with an elevated international normalized ration (INR) level. Which of the following would be ordered as the antidote for warfarin?
    1. Vitamin K
    2. Vitamin B$_{12}$
    3. Calcium chloride
    4. Protamine sulfate

18. Which of the following is a desired outcome for the nursing diagnosis of *Acute Pain* for a patient with acute thrombophlebitis?
    1. States anxiety is decreased.
    2. States pain is satisfactorily relieved.
    3. Is able to participate in desired activities.
    4. Reports ability to ambulate without pain.

19. A patient visits the doctor for a severe sore throat and fever. As the nurse plans the patient's care, which of the following diagnostic tests is obtained to prevent cardiac complications?
    1. Chest x-ray examination
    2. Throat culture
    3. White blood cell count
    4. Erythrocyte sedimentation rate

20. The nurse is reviewing the daily international normalized ration (INR) and prothrombin time (PT) levels for a patient who had a mechanical valve replacement. The INR is 3.7 and the PT level is 29. Which of the following actions should the nurse take?
    1. Give the next dose of warfarin (Coumadin) as ordered.
    2. Inform the health care provider now.
    3. Give warfarin (Coumadin) now.
    4. Hold the next dose of warfarin (Coumadin).

21. A patient, who had a hysterectomy 2 days ago, reports tenderness in her left calf. The nursing assessment reveals the following: left calf 17.5", right calf 14", left thigh 32", right thigh 28", and a shiny, warm, and reddened left leg. Which of the following interventions should be given priority in the patient's plan of care? **Select all that apply.**
    1. Maintain bedrest.
    2. Encourage ambulation three times daily.
    3. Encourage bilateral leg exercises.
    4. Apply bilateral antiembolism stockings.
    5. Apply right antiembolism stocking.
    6. Apply warm moist heat as ordered.

22. Which of the following findings should be reported to the physician for a patient receiving warfarin therapy?
    1. Bleeding time 3 (normal = 2–5 seconds)
    2. International normalized ratio (INR) 4 (therapeutic = 2–3 seconds)
    3. Partial thromboplastin time (PTT) 28 (normal = 30–45 seconds)
    4. Prothrombin time (PT) 20 (therapeutic = 13.5–22 seconds)

23. A patient who has end-stage dilated cardiomyopathy comes to the emergency department with dyspnea. The patient reports waking with a feeling of suffocation, which was frightening. Which of the following responses by the nurse is most appropriate?
    1. "You must have been dreaming."
    2. "Reclining decreases the heart's ability to pump blood."
    3. "Sleeping increases heart rate, which increases the body's need for oxygen."
    4. "Reclining increases fluid returning to the heart, which builds up fluid in the lungs."

24. Which of the following assessments of a patient would indicate a side effect of digoxin (Lanoxin) is occurring that requires follow-up?
    1. Skin flushing
    2. Anorexia
    3. Hypertension
    4. Constipation

25. The physician writes a "now" order for codeine 45 mg intramuscular (IM) for a patient with thrombophlebitis. The nurse has on hand codeine 60 mg/2 mL. Which of the following doses should be given?
    1. 1.45 mL
    2. 1.5 mL
    3. 1.75 mL
    4. 2.15 mL

26. A patient, age 46, is admitted for observation with a chest contusion after hitting the steering wheel in an auto accident. Which of the following findings would be the highest priority?
    1. Bronchovesicular sounds heard over the major airways
    2. Patient reports chest soreness and tenderness
    3. Sternal bruising noted
    4. Pericardial rub heard on auscultation

24

Nursing Care of Patients With Occlusive Cardiovascular Disorders

VOCABULARY

Match the term with its definition.

1. _____ Lymphangitis
2. _____ Atherosclerosis
3. _____ Stenosis
4. _____ Ischemia
5. _____ Venous stasis ulcer
6. _____ High-density lipoprotein
7. _____ Collateral circulation
8. _____ Balloon angioplasty
9. _____ Chest pain caused by decreased blood supply to the heart
10. _____ Chest pain that usually subsides with rest
11. _____ Chest pain that increases in frequency and is not relieved by rest
12. _____ Tortuous and bulging veins, usually in lower extremity
13. _____ Disease-causing venospasms when exposed to cold
14. _____ A bulging or dilation of an artery
15. _____ Death of a portion of the myocardium
16. _____ Laboratory value that determines degree of damage to the heart
17. _____ Embolism
18. _____ Thrombus
19. _____ Intermittent claudication
20. _____ Coronary artery disease

1. Varicose veins
2. Procedure that compresses plaque against wall of artery
3. Unstable angina
4. Bacterial infection of lymphatic channels
5. Angina pectoris
6. Obstructed blood flow in the coronary arteries
7. Stable angina
8. Raynaud's disease
9. Plaque buildup within arterial wall
10. Lack of sufficient blood supply
11. Aneurysm
12. Vessels grow to compensate for blocked blood flow
13. Narrowing of a vessel
14. Myocardial infarction
15. A moving clot
16. "Good" cholesterol
17. A stationary clot
18. Skin breakdown from chronic venous insufficiency
19. Troponin I
20. Exertional calf pain that ceases with rest

ATHEROSCLEROSIS

Answer the following questions.

1. What is the pathophysiology of atherosclerosis?

_____

_____

2. What are modifiable risk factors that contribute to atherosclerosis?

_____

_____

3. Develop a teaching plan for one of the modifiable risk factors for atherosclerosis.

_____

_____

MYOCARDIAL INFARCTION

Find the 22 errors and insert the correct information.

Myocardial infarction (MI) is the death of a portion of the pericardial sac caused by blockage or spasm of a coronary artery. When the patient has an MI, the affected part of the muscle becomes damaged and no longer functions properly. Ischemic injury takes a few minutes before complete necrosis and infarction take place. The ischemic process affects the subendocardial layer, which is the least sensitive to hypoxia. Myocardial contractility is depressed, so the body attempts to compensate by triggering the parasympathetic nervous system. This causes a decrease in myocardial oxygen demand, which further depresses the myocardium. After necrosis, the contractility function of the muscle is temporarily lost. If treatment is initiated after several signs of an MI, the area of damage can be minimized. If prolonged ischemia occurs, the size of the infarction can be small.

The area that is affected by an MI depends on which coronary artery is involved. The left anterior descending (LAD) branch of the left main coronary artery is the area that feeds the lateral wall. The right coronary artery (RCA) feeds the anterior wall and parts of the atrioventricular node and the sinoatrial node. An occlusion of the RCA leads to an inferior MI and to abnormalities of impulse conduction and formation. The left circumflex coronary artery feeds the inferior wall and part of the posterior wall of the heart.

Pain is the least common symptom. The pain does not radiate. The patient usually believes that an MI is occurring. Other symptoms may include restlessness, a feeling of impending doom, nausea, diaphoresis, and cold, clammy, ashen skin. The only symptom that might be present in the older adult is vomiting. Women may have atypical symptoms of an MI.

The three strong indicators of an MI are patient history, abnormal electrocardiographic (ECG) readings, and high triglyceride levels.

Initially, patients are kept on bedrest to increase myocardial oxygen demand. Patients are medicated promptly when experiencing chest pain. Meperidine (Demerol) is the most widely used narcotic for MI. It helps decrease anxiety, increases respirations, and vasoconstricts the coronary arteries. Oxygen is given usually at 1 L/hr via nasal cannula. Nitroglycerin sublingual, topical, or by intravenous (IV) drip can also be administered. Percutaneous coronary intervention is a frequent treatment option for an occluded coronary artery.

A nursing care plan should include factors that may contribute to decreased cardiac workload. Changes in diet, stress reduction, regular exercise program, smoking cessation, and following a medication schedule require extensive patient and family teaching.

PHARMACOLOGICAL TREATMENT

Match the medication to the appropriate description.

1. _____ Calcium channel blocker
2. _____ Beta blocker
3. _____ Drug of choice for anginal attacks
4. _____ Does not dissolve existing clots
5. _____ Bile acid sequestrant
6. _____ Antiplatelet
7. _____ Long-acting nitrate
8. _____ Thrombolytic therapy agent
9. _____ Decreases blood viscosity
10. _____ Reduces cholesterol synthesis

1. Nitroglycerin
2. Cholestyramine (Questran)
3. Propranolol (Inderal)
4. Amlodipine (Norvasc)
5. Reteplase (Retavase)
6. Clopidogrel (Plavix)
7. Heparin
8. Pentoxifylline (Trental)
9. Isosorbide dinitrate (Isordil)
10. Atorvastatin (Lipitor)

CRITICAL THINKING

Read the following case study and answer the questions.

Mr. Edwards is a 43-year-old man with a history of peripheral vascular disease and hypertension. He smokes two packs of cigarettes per day. He reports calf pain during minimal exercise that decreases with rest.

1. Which of the following nursing diagnoses would be the most appropriate relating to Mr. Edwards's symptoms, and what would be the patient outcome? _____

_____

_____

A. *Ineffective Tissue Perfusion* related to compromised circulation

B. *Fatigue* related to pain on exertion

C. *Impaired Mobility* relating to stress associated with pain

D. *Self-Care Deficit* related to pain and muscle spasms

2. Explain what happens when intermittent claudication occurs. _____
_____
_____

3. Why does rest decrease the pain? _____
_____
_____

4. Describe how smoking contributes to decreased circulation. _____
_____
_____

REVIEW QUESTIONS—CONTENT REVIEW

Choose the best answer unless directed otherwise.

1. Before a cardiac catheterization and coronary arteriogram, it is essential that the nurse ask a patient if the patient is allergic to which of the following?
   1. Eggs
   2. Codeine
   3. Iodine
   4. Penicillin

2. A patient, hospitalized with an MI, suddenly begins having severe respiratory distress with frothy sputum. These signs indicate that the patient probably has developed which of the following?
   1. Pneumonia
   2. Cardiac tamponade
   3. Pulmonary edema
   4. Pneumothorax

3. As the nurse examines a patient for decreased circulation in the lower extremities, which of the following findings would indicate adequate circulation?
   1. Loss of hair on the extremity
   2. Capillary refill less than 3 seconds
   3. Diminished pulses in the extremity
   4. Thickened nails of the extremity

4. The nurse is teaching the patient about diet. Which of the following dietary actions may reduce low-density lipid (LDL) cholesterol?
   1. Consuming <5 grams of soluble fiber daily
   2. Consuming >200 mg cholesterol daily
   3. <7% Kcal as saturated fat
   4. Using whole milk

5. The nurse understands that pain associated with coronary artery disease occurs from which of the following?
   1. Lack of nutrients to the heart
   2. Interrupted electrical activity to the areas of the heart
   3. Lack of sufficient oxygen to the myocardium
   4. Overexertion of heart muscle due to the workload

REVIEW QUESTIONS—TEST PREPARATION

Choose the best answer unless directed otherwise.

6. A patient who has been scheduled for a stress electrocardiogram (ECG) asks why this ECG is needed. Which of the following is the nurse's best response?
   1. "It can predict whether the patient may soon have a heart attack."
   2. "It verifies how much more physically fit the patient needs to become."
   3. "It determines the patient's potential target heart rate."
   4. "It shows how the heart performs during exercise."

7. During a stress ECG, a patient reports chest pain, and the test is stopped. When the patient is asked to undergo a heart catheterization, the patient appears apprehensive and worried. Which of the following is the most appropriate action for the nurse to take to reduce the patient's anxiety?
   1. Explain how coronary artery disease is treated.
   2. Avoid discussing the heart catheterization until the patient has relaxed.
   3. Explain how well others have done after having this procedure.
   4. Listen to the patient express feelings about the situation.

8. Which of the following statements by a patient demonstrates to the nurse that the patient understands when to replace nitroglycerin tablets?
   1. Pills no longer cause tingling sensation when used.
   2. Pills disintegrate when touched.
   3. Pills smell like vinegar.
   4. Pills become discolored.

9. After hospitalization for a myocardial infarction, a patient is placed on a low-sodium diet. In discussing foods allowed on this diet, the nurse should inform the patient that this list includes which of the following?
   1. Hot dogs
   2. Fresh vegetables
   3. Milk and cheese
   4. Canned soups

10. Which of the following does the nurse correctly include in a teaching plan as modifiable risk factors for coronary artery disease? **Select all that apply.**
    1. Hypertension
    2. Gender
    3. Age
    4. Smoking
    5. Diabetes

11. Which of the following should the nurse correctly include in a teaching plan as being high in saturated fat? **Select all that apply.**
    1. Avocado
    2. Tuna fish
    3. Beef
    4. Olive oil
    5. Poultry
    6. Coconut oil

12. The nurse is collecting data on a patient. Which of the following clinical manifestations would the nurse expect to find with acute venous insufficiency? **Select all that apply.**
    1. Full superficial veins
    2. An aching, cramping type of pain
    3. Initial absence of edema
    4. Cool and cyanotic skin
    5. Positive Homans' sign
    6. Hyperemia

13. The nurse understands that which of the following are the most characteristic symptoms of Buerger's disease? **Select all that apply.**
    1. Numbness
    2. Pain
    3. Cramping
    4. Swelling
    5. Bounding pulses
    6. Intermittent claudication

14. A patient has been diagnosed with Raynaud's disease and asks the nurse what occurs with this disease. Which of the following is the most appropriate response?
    1. "Arterial vessel occlusion is caused by many clots that develop in the heart and are carried to the bloodstream."
    2. "Arteriolar vasoconstriction occurs, most often in the fingertips with symptoms of coldness, pain, and pale skin."
    3. "Peripheral vasospasm occurs in the lower limbs as a result of valve damage from long-standing venous stasis."
    4. "Thrombosis related to prolonged vasoconstriction caused by overexposure to the cold occurs."

VOCABULARY

Match the words and definitions.

1. _____ Amplitude
2. _____ Atrial depolarization
3. _____ Atrial systole
4. _____ Bigeminy
5. _____ Cardioversion
6. _____ Complete heart block
7. _____ Contractility
8. _____ Decompensation
9. _____ Defibrillate
10. _____ Inherent
11. _____ Ischemia
12. _____ Isoelectric line
13. _____ Multifocal
14. _____ Quadrigeminy
15. _____ Right bundle branch block
16. _____ Trigeminy
17. _____ Unifocal
18. _____ Ventricular diastole
19. _____ Ventricular escape rhythm
20. _____ Ventricular repolarization
21. _____ Ventricular systole

1. Beat occurring every fourth complex, as in premature ventricular contractions (PVCs)
2. Belonging to anything naturally
3. Coming or originating from one site
4. Condition in which there is a complete dissociation between atrial and ventricular systoles
5. Contraction of the atria
6. Contraction of the two ventricles
7. Defect in heart conduction system in which right bundle does not conduct impulses normally
8. Elective procedure in which synchronized shock of 25 to 50 joules is delivered to restore normal sinus rhythm
9. Electrical activation of the atria
10. Electrical tracing is at zero and is neither positive nor negative
11. Failure of the heart to maintain adequate circulation
12. Force with which left ventricular ejection occurs
13. Local deficiency of blood supply resulting from obstruction of the circulation to another part
14. Occurring every third beat, as in PVCs
15. Occurs every second beat, as in PVCs
16. Originating from many foci or sites
17. Period of relaxation of the ventricle
18. Reestablishment of the polarized state of the muscle after contraction
19. Size or fullness of voltage
20. Naturally occurring rhythm of the ventricles when the rest of the conduction system fails
21. Use of electrical device to apply countershocks to the heart through electrodes placed on the chest wall to stop fibrillation

COMPONENTS OF A CARDIAC CYCLE

Label the components of a cardiac cycle.

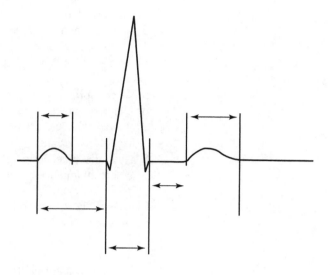

HEART RATE

Calculate the heart rate using the 6-second method.

1.

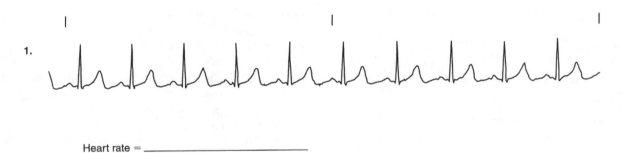

Heart rate = _____

2.

Heart rate = _____

3.

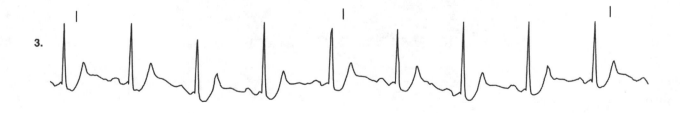

Heart rate = _____

CARDIAC CONDUCTION

Match the words and definitions.

1. _____ Sinoatrial node
2. _____ Atrioventricular node
3. _____ Normal sinus rhythm
4. _____ Right atrium
5. _____ Right ventricle
6. _____ Left atrium
7. _____ Left ventricle
8. _____ Bradycardia
9. _____ Tachycardia
10. _____ Q wave
11. _____ P wave
12. _____ R wave
13. _____ S wave
14. _____ T wave
15. _____ U wave
16. _____ Premature
17. _____ Sinus tachycardia
18. _____ Sinus bradycardia
19. _____ Premature atrial contraction
20. _____ Atrial fibrillation
21. _____ Premature ventricular contraction
22. _____ Ventricular tachycardia
23. _____ Ventricular fibrillation
24. _____ Asystole

1. Rate less than 60
2. No QRS complexes seen—straight line
3. An early beat
4. An early beat that has a P wave and a normal QRS complex
5. Where normal cardiac impulse originates
6. A chaotic pattern—no visible cardiac cycles
7. No identifiable P waves with a normal QRS complex; irregularly irregular
8. Wave that precedes a QRS complex
9. Where an impulse is delayed before going to the Purkinje fibers
10. An early beat with no P wave and a wide, bizarre QRS complex
11. Successive beats of three or more wide, bizarre QRS complexes
12. Rhythm with normal P waves, QRS, T waves with a heart rate of 60 to 100 beats per minute
13. The first negative deflection of a QRS complex
14. A small wave seen after the T wave
15. The first positive deflection on a QRS complex
16. Rhythm with normal P waves, QRS, T waves with a heart rate of less than 60 beats per minute
17. The chamber of the heart that pumps the blood to the rest of the body
18. The chamber that receives blood returning to the heart
19. Rhythm with normal P waves, QRS, T waves with a heart rate of more than 100 beats per minute
20. The wave that follows the QRS complex
21. The chamber that receives blood from the pulmonary veins
22. The downward deflection after the R wave
23. Heart rate of more than 100 beats per minute
24. Chamber that propels blood into the pulmonary artery

ELECTROCARDIOGRAM INTERPRETATION

Analyze the electrocardiogram (ECG) rhythms using the six-step interpretation process.

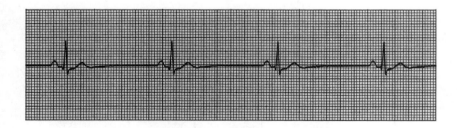

A.

1. Rhythm: _____

2. Heart rate: _____

3. P waves: _____

4. PR interval: _____

5. QRS interval: _____

6. QT interval: _____

7. ECG interpretation: _____

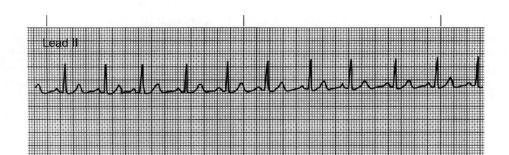

B.

1. Rhythm: _____

2. Heart rate: _____

3. P waves: _____

4. PR interval: _____

5. QRS interval: _____

6. QT interval: _____

7. ECG interpretation: _____

CRITICAL THINKING

Read the following case study and answer the questions.

Mrs. Samuels is admitted to the hospital for chest pain. Tests are run, and her electrocardiogram (ECG) shows bigeminal PVCs of more than 6 per minute that are close to her T wave. Her potassium level is 2.8 mEq/L. She is short of breath on exertion. Her blood pressure is 104/56 mm Hg, pulse is 72 beats per minute, and respirations are 16 per minute.

1. What should the nurse do first? _____

_____

_____

2. What actions should the nurse take regarding the dysrhythmia? _____

_____

3. What might some of the causes be for this dysrhythmia?

_____

_____

4. What additional symptoms might the nurse anticipate?

_____

_____

5. What type of orders should the nurse expect from the health care provider? _____

_____

REVIEW QUESTIONS—CONTENT REVIEW

Choose the best answer unless directed otherwise.

1. The nurse understands that which of the following defines a cardiac cycle?
   1. Circulation of the blood through the body
   2. Circulation of the blood through the heart
   3. Depolarization and repolarization of heart chambers
   4. Pumping action of the heart

2. The heart receives blood returning from the body through which of the following?
   1. Pulmonary vein
   2. Aorta
   3. Vena cavae
   4. Right coronary artery

3. Which of the following separates the right side of the heart from the left?
   1. Chamber
   2. Pericardium
   3. Valve
   4. Septum

4. Which of the following chambers of the heart is largest and has the thickest myocardium?
   1. Left ventricle
   2. Right ventricle
   3. Right atrium
   4. Left atrium

5. Which of the following waveforms represents the resting state of the ventricle on the ECG?
   1. P wave
   2. QRS complex
   3. U wave
   4. T wave

6. Which of the following is the normal rate for the sinoatrial node?
   1. 20 to 40 beats per minute
   2. 40 to 60 beats per minute
   3. 60 to 100 beats per minute
   4. More than 100 beats per minute

7. The nurse understands that rhythms arising from the primary pacing node of the heart are referred to as which of the following?
   1. Escape beats
   2. Bundle branch blocks
   3. Sinus rhythms
   4. Ectopic rhythms

REVIEW QUESTIONS—TEST PREPARATION

Choose the best answer unless directed otherwise.

8. The nurse notes a life-threatening dysrhythmia on a patient's cardiac monitor. Which of the following is the nurse's first appropriate action?
   1. Notify the health care provider immediately.
   2. Assess the patient.
   3. Administer the appropriate medication for the noted dysrhythmia.
   4. Obtain vital signs.

9. The nurse is teaching a patient about digoxin. Which of the following should the nurse include in the teaching?
   1. Digoxin decreases ectopic beats.
   2. The force of contractions is increased with digoxin.
   3. The resting heart rate increases when digoxin is taken.
   4. Digoxin raises the resting blood pressure.

10. The nurse is providing care to a patient with atrial fibrillation. Which of the following statements, if made by the patient, would be of the most concern?
    1. "Aspirin upsets my stomach, so I quit taking it."
    2. "It seems like my feet are a little swollen."
    3. "My wife and I got a membership at the local health club."
    4. "I've been having trouble falling asleep at night."

11. Which of the following treatments can be appropriate for a patient with atrial fibrillation? **Select all that apply.**
    1. Amiodarone (Cordarone)
    2. Nitroglycerin
    3. Warfarin (Coumadin)
    4. Digoxin (Lanoxin)
    5. Cardioversion
    6. Epinephrine

12. The nurse is caring for a patient who has had a run of three or more PVCs together. The nurse should document this as which of the following?
    1. Ventricular tachycardia
    2. Bigeminy
    3. Trigeminy
    4. Multifocal PVCs

13. The nurse is caring for a patient in ventricular tachycardia who is hemodynamically stable. Which of the following is the initial treatment for this dysrhythmia?
    1. Cardioversion
    2. Pacemaker
    3. Defibrillation
    4. Antiarrhythmic intravenous (IV) medication

14. The nurse is caring for a patient whose ECG monitor shows a total absence of electrical impulse. The nurse does not detect a pulse. The nurse would document this as which of the following rhythms?
    1. Agonal
    2. Asystole
    3. Sinus arrest
    4. Ventricular standstill

15. A patient with a cardiac disorder is having increased PVCs and feels "anxious." After assessment and vital signs, what is the next action for the nurse to take?
    1. Order an ECG and cardiac enzymes.
    2. Call the health care provider.
    3. Elevate the head of the bed and start oxygen at 2 L/min.
    4. Put the bed in modified Trendelenburg's position.

16. The nurse is caring for a patient who is fatigued and undergoing cardiac testing. For which of the following dysrhythmias will the nurse anticipate the patient's need for a permanent pacemaker? **Select all that apply.**
    1. Ventricular fibrillation
    2. First-degree heart block
    3. Atrial fibrillation
    4. Third-degree heart block
    5. Symptomatic bradycardia
    6. Premature atrial contractions (PACs)

26 Nursing Care of Patients With Heart Failure

VOCABULARY

Fill in the blank with the appropriate word found in the word list.

Afterload   Peripheral vascular resistance

Cor pulmonale   Preload

Hepatomegaly   Pulmonary edema (acute heart failure)

Orthopnea   Splenomegaly

Paroxysmal nocturnal dyspnea

1. _____ is the acute inability of the heart to pump enough blood to meet the body's oxygen and nutrient needs.

2. _____ occurs when the right side of the heart fails because of an increased workload caused by pulmonary disease.

3. Organ enlargement that may occur with right-sided heart failure (HF) is known as _____ and _____.

4. The goal of treatment for HF is to improve the heart's pumping ability and decrease the heart's workload by reducing _____.

5. _____ causes supine patients to awaken suddenly with a feeling of suffocation.

6. The end-diastole stretch in the ventricles produced by ventricular volume is _____.

7. The tension in the ventricular wall during systole necessary to overcome vascular resistance is _____.

8. _____ is dyspnea that occurs when the patient lies down.

FLUID ACCUMULATION PATTERNS

Label the backward accumulation of fluid and shade areas of fluid congestion.

The heart pumps blood in a closed circuit. If one side of the heart fails to adequately pump blood forward, it pools and backs up from the failing chamber. On the drawing, use arrows to mark the path of the backward accumulation of fluid from the side of the heart that is failing. Shade in areas where fluid congestion occurs.

To increase your understanding of where the backward accumulation of fluid occurs from a certain side of the heart, use blue shading to illustrate the side with deoxygenated blood accumulation. Use red shading for the side with oxygenated blood accumulation.

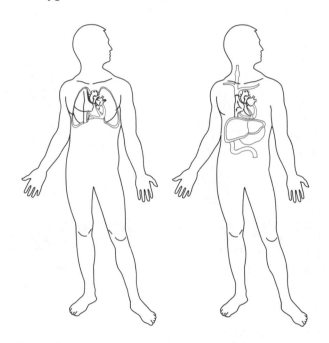

SIGNS AND SYMPTOMS OF HEART FAILURE

In HF, certain signs and symptoms occur based on the side of the heart that is failing as a pump.

Match the following sign or symptom to the failing side of the heart that is causing it.

1. _____ Dry cough
2. _____ Peripheral edema
3. _____ Crackles
4. _____ Hepatomegaly
5. _____ Jugular vein distention
6. _____ Dyspnea
7. _____ Splenomegaly
8. _____ Orthopnea

1. Left-sided HF
2. Right-sided HF

CRITICAL THINKING

Read the following case study and answer the questions.

Mr. Donner, age 72, is admitted to the cardiac unit for increasing dyspnea on exertion and fatigue.

Subjective Data
History of HF for 2 years
Unable to walk one block without increasing dyspnea
Sleeps at 60-degree angle in reclining chair
Increasing fatigue during the last 2 weeks

Objective Data
BP 140/78 mm Hg, P 108 beats per minute, R 24 per minute, T 98.8°F (37.1°C)
Jugular vein distention at 45 degrees
Has frequent dry cough
Bilateral crackles in lung bases
Nonpitting edema
Diagnostic studies
Chest x-ray examination: left and right ventricular hypertrophy, bilateral fluid in lower lung lobes

1. Explain the cause of Mr. Donner's fatigue, cough, and shortness of breath. _____

_____

2. Which of Mr. Donner's signs and symptoms are from left-sided HF and which are from right-sided HF?
   Left: _____
   Right: _____

_____

3. Explain the purpose of each of the following therapies. How would they be beneficial in treating Mr. Donner's heart failure?
   1. Furosemide (Lasix) 40 mg by mouth (PO) twice daily: _____
   2. Benazepril (Lotensin) 10 mg PO daily: _____

_____

   3. 2 g sodium diet: _____
   4. Oxygen 4 L/min: _____

_____

4. Mr. Donner suddenly becomes dyspneic and anxious, has moist crackles throughout his lungs, and pink frothy sputum. Explain what is happening. _____

_____

5. Explain the purpose of each of the following therapies. How are they beneficial in treating Mr. Donner's acute HF? _____

   1. High Fowler's position: _____

   _____

   2. Oxygen 6 L/min: _____

   _____

   3. Furosemide (Lasix) intravenous push (IVP): _____

   _____

   4. Nitroglycerin IV infusion: _____

   _____

   5. Morphine 2 mg IVP: _____

   _____

6. List two priority nursing diagnoses and goals for Mr. Donner's chronic HF.

   _____

   _____

   _____

   _____

   _____

   _____

7. What are Mr. Donner's health learning needs to manage his chronic condition?

   _____

   _____

   _____

   _____

   _____

   _____

REVIEW QUESTIONS—CONTENT REVIEW

Choose the best answer unless directed otherwise.

1. A patient is being given digoxin (Lanoxin) to treat heart failure. Which of the following is a usual adult daily dosage of digoxin (Lanoxin)?
   1. 0.005 mg
   2. 0.025 mg
   3. 0.25 mg
   4. 2.5 mg

2. When the nurse is reviewing a patient's daily laboratory test results, which of the following electrolyte imbalances should the nurse recognize as predisposing the patient to digoxin toxicity?
   1. Hypokalemia
   2. Hyperkalemia
   3. Hyponatremia
   4. Hypernatremia

3. If a patient has elevated pulmonary vascular pressures, the nurse understands that the patient is most likely to develop which of the following physiological cardiac changes?
   1. Left atrial atrophy
   2. Right atrial atrophy
   3. Left ventricular hypertrophy
   4. Right ventricular hypertrophy

REVIEW QUESTIONS—TEST PREPARATION

Choose the best answer unless directed otherwise.

4. A patient is admitted to a medical unit with a diagnosis of heart failure. The patient reports increasing fatigue during the past 2 weeks. Which of the following is the most likely cause of this fatigue?
   1. Dyspnea
   2. Decreased cardiac output
   3. Dry cough
   4. Orthopnea

5. A patient asks the nurse what a diagnosis of heart failure means. Which of the following is the nurse's best response?
   1. "Your heart briefly stops."
   2. "Your heart has an area of muscle that is dead."
   3. "Your heart is pumping too much blood."
   4. "Your heart is not an efficient pump."

6. A patient's chest x-ray examination indicates fluid in both lung bases. Which of the following signs or symptoms present during the nurse's data collection most reflects these x-ray examination findings?
   1. Fatigue
   2. Peripheral edema
   3. Bilateral crackles
   4. Jugular vein distention

7. To monitor the severity of a patient's heart failure, which of the following information is the most appropriate for the nurse to gather daily?
   1. Weight
   2. Calorie count
   3. Appetite
   4. Abdominal girth

8. Which of the following signs indicates to the nurse that digoxin (Lanoxin) has been effective for a patient?
   1. Urine output decreases
   2. Urine output increases
   3. Heart rate higher than 95 beats per minute
   4. Heart rate lower than 50 beats per minute

9. For a patient who is being discharged on digoxin (Lanoxin), the nurse should include which of the following in an explanation to the patient on the signs and symptoms of digoxin toxicity?
   1. Poor appetite
   2. Constipation
   3. Halos around lights
   4. Tachycardia

10. The patient is being discharged on furosemide (Lasix). The nurse evaluates the patient as understanding medication teaching if the patient states that which of the following laboratory tests will be monitored as ordered?
    1. "I will have my urine sodium checked."
    2. "I will have my calcium level checked."
    3. "I will have my prothrombin time checked."
    4. "I will have my potassium level checked."

11. Which of the following does the nurse understand are the reasons a patient with pulmonary edema is given morphine sulfate? **Select all that apply.**
    1. To reduce anxiety
    2. To relieve chest pain
    3. To strengthen heart contractions
    4. To increase blood pressure
    5. To reduce preload and afterload
    6. To induce amnesia

12. The nurse evaluates that bumetanide (Bumex) IV is effective in treating pulmonary edema if which of the following patient signs or symptoms is resolved?
    1. Pedal edema
    2. Jugular venous distention
    3. Pink, frothy sputum
    4. Bradycardia

13. A patient is being taught the action of digoxin, which is an inotropic agent. The nurse defines an inotropic agent as a medication that has which of the following actions?
    1. Decreases heart rate.
    2. Increases heart rate.
    3. Increases conduction time.
    4. Strengthens heart contraction.

14. For a patient receiving furosemide, the nurse evaluates the medication as being effective if which of the following effects occurs?
    1. Bilateral crackles diminish.
    2. Serum potassium decreases.
    3. Heart rate increases.
    4. Pulse pressure increases.

15. When caring for an anxious patient with dyspnea, which of the following nursing actions is most helpful to include in the plan of care to relieve anxiety?
    1. Increase activity levels.
    2. Stay at patient's bedside.
    3. Pull the privacy curtain.
    4. Close the patient's door.

unit SIX

Understanding the Hematologic and Lymphatic Systems

CHECKLIST FOR LEARNING SUCCESS

Review of Anatomy and Physiology and Aging Changes	Major Disorders	Nursing Assessment	Diagnostic Tests	Interventions	Common Medications
❏ Blood components	❏ Anemias	❏ Signs and symptoms of anemias	❏ Complete blood cell count (CBC)	❏ Blood product administration	❏ Iron
❏ Functions of different blood cells	❏ Polycythemia	❏ Signs and symptoms of bleeding	❏ White blood cell (WBC) differential	❏ Chemotherapy	❏ Colony-stimulating factors
❏ Lymphatic system structures and functions	❏ Disseminated intravascular coagulation	❏ Lymph nodes	❏ Coagulation tests	❏ Thrombocytopenia precautions	❏ Chemotherapy
❏ Effects of aging	❏ Idiopathic thrombocytopenic purpura	❏ Skin	❏ Bone marrow biopsy	❏ Infection precautions	❏ Clotting factors
	❏ Hemophilia		❏ Lymphangiography	❏ Bone marrow transplant	
	❏ Leukemias		❏ Lymph node biopsy	❏ Splenectomy	
	❏ Multiple myeloma				
	❏ Hodgkin's disease				
	❏ Lymphomas				
	❏ Spleen disorders				

27

Hematologic and Lymphatic System Function, Assessment, and Therapeutic Measures

VOCABULARY

Fill in the blank with the appropriate word.

1. _____ is a blue-black discoloration from hemorrhage under the skin.

2. _____ is the term used to describe swelling from blockage of lymph circulation.

3. Tiny hemorrhages into the skin creating a polka-dot appearance are called _____.

4. _____ is caused by hemorrhages into the skin, mucous membranes, or internal organs.

5. The patient with _____ has an increased risk for bleeding because of insufficient platelets.

LYMPHATIC SYSTEM REVIEW

Match each part of the lymphatic system with its proper description.

1. _____ Lymph capillaries

2. _____ Lymph nodules

3. _____ Thoracic duct

4. _____ Lymph nodes

5. _____ Valves

1. Destroy pathogens in the lymph from the extremities before the lymph is returned to the blood

2. Collect tissue fluid from intercellular spaces

3. Prevent backflow of lymph in larger lymph vessels

4. Destroy pathogens that penetrate mucous membranes

5. Empties lymph from the lower body and upper left quadrant into the left subclavian vein

STRUCTURES OF THE LYMPHATIC SYSTEM

Label the following structures.

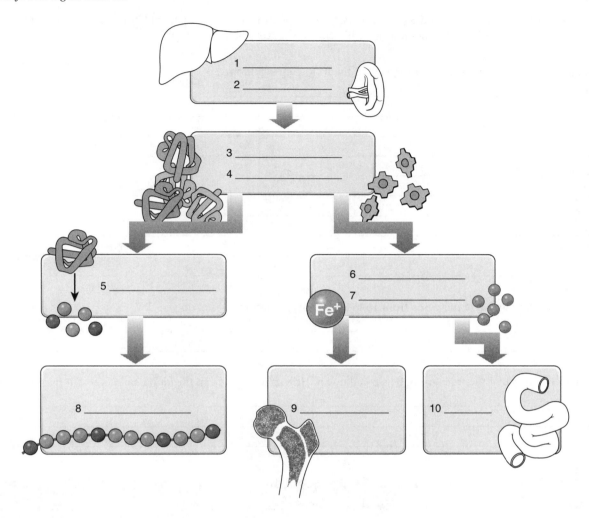

1. _____
2. _____
3. _____
4. _____
5. _____
6. _____
7. _____
8. _____
9. _____
10. _____

HEMATOLOGIC SYSTEM REVIEW

Match each term with its definition.

1. _____ Albumin
2. _____ Macrophages
3. _____ Calcium ions
4. _____ Intrinsic factor
5. _____ Hemoglobin
6. _____ Basophils
7. _____ Red bone marrow
8. _____ Stem cell
9. _____ Megakaryocyte
10. _____ Lymphocytes

1. May become any kind of blood cell
2. Essential for chemical clotting
3. Release histamine
4. A hematopoietic tissue
5. May become cells that produce antibodies
6. Large phagocytic cells
7. Promotes absorption of vitamin B_{12}
8. Its fragments become platelets
9. Carries oxygen in red blood cells (RBCs)
10. Pulls tissue fluid into capillaries to maintain blood volume

CRITICAL THINKING

Read the case study and answer the questions.

Mr. Foster is receiving a unit of packed RBCs. You assist with identification of the patient before the transfusion begins. The registered nurse (RN) then delegates monitoring of his vital signs every half hour to you.

1. Why should Mr. Foster be monitored for each of the following symptoms?

   1. Fever _____

   _____

   2. Back pain _____

   _____

   3. Respiratory distress _____

   _____

   4. Crackles _____

   _____

   5. Hives _____

   _____

2. Mr. Foster's respiratory rate increases from 16 to 20 breaths per minute. What do you do?

   _____

   _____

3. The physician asks that the transfusion be slowed down. How many hours can the blood hang before it must be stopped?

   _____

   _____

   _____

REVIEW QUESTIONS—CONTENT REVIEW

Choose the best answer unless directed otherwise.

1. What is the mineral necessary for chemical clotting?
   1. Iron
   2. Sodium
   3. Potassium
   4. Calcium

2. Through which of the following does lymph return to the blood?
   1. Carotid arteries
   2. Aorta
   3. Inferior vena cava
   4. Subclavian veins

3. Which of the following is a normal hemoglobin value?
   1. 38% to 48%
   2. 12 to 18 g/100 mL
   3. 48 to 54 mg %
   4. 27 to 36 g/dL

4. Which laboratory study is monitored for the patient receiving heparin therapy?
   1. International normalized ratio (INR)
   2. Prothrombin time (PT)
   3. Partial thromboplastin time (PTT)
   4. Bleeding time

5. Which blood product replaces missing clotting factors in the patient who has a bleeding disorder?
   1. Platelets
   2. Packed RBCs
   3. Albumin
   4. Cryoprecipitate

6. Which of the following items are transported in blood plasma? **Select all that apply.**
   1. Oxygen
   2. Nutrients
   3. Carbon dioxide
   4. Hormones
   5. Wastes
   6. Electrolytes

Choose the best answer unless directed otherwise.

7. A patient is on warfarin (Coumadin) therapy and has an INR of 1.6. Which action by the nurse is appropriate?
   1. Observe the patient for abnormal bleeding.
   2. Notify the physician and expect an order to increase the warfarin dose.
   3. Advise the patient to double today's dose of warfarin.
   4. Administer vitamin K per protocol.

8. A patient receiving a transfusion of packed RBCs reports chest and back pain. How should the nurse respond?
   1. Do a complete head-to-toe examination.
   2. Ask the patient to rate the pain on a 0 to 10 scale.
   3. Stop the transfusion and call the RN stat depending on agency policy.
   4. Administer an analgesic, as needed (prn).

9. The nurse is preparing to assist the physician with a bone marrow biopsy. Which of the following interventions is most important for the nurse to carry out before the procedure?
   1. Explain the procedure to the patient's family.
   2. Administer an analgesic to the patient.
   3. Observe the patient for bleeding.
   4. Drape the biopsy site.

10. The nurse is providing care for patients on a medical surgical unit. Which of the following patients is at increased risk for infection?
    1. A 57-year-old whose WBC count = 6500/mm^3
    2. A 63-year-old with a platelet count = 110,000/mm^3
    3. A 49-year-old with a hematocrit = 44%
    4. An 88-year-old with a neutrophil count of 32%

28

Nursing Care of Patients With Hematologic and Lymphatic Disorders

VOCABULARY

Label each statement true or false.

1. _____ Anemia is a reduction in white blood cells (WBCs).
2. _____ Hemolysis is the destruction of red blood cells (RBCs).
3. _____ Pancytopenia is reduced numbers of all blood cells.
4. _____ Polycythemia is the production of excess blood cells.
5. _____ Phlebotomy is the excision of a vessel.
6. _____ Disseminated intravascular coagulation (DIC) involves accelerated clotting throughout the circulation.
7. _____ Thrombocytopenia is an increase in platelets.
8. _____ Hemarthrosis is bleeding into the muscles.
9. _____ Leukemia literally means "white blood."
10. _____ Cancer of the lymph system is called lymphemia.
11. _____ Abnormalities in B cells and T cells can result in lymphoma
12. _____ Enlargement of the spleen is called splenomegaly.

CRITICAL THINKING: LEUKEMIA

Read the case study and answer the questions.

Mr. Frantzis is a 60-year-old man in the acute stage of chronic lymphocytic leukemia. He is admitted to a nursing home because he has no family to help care for him. He has had chemotherapy in the past but has decided against further treatment. You are assigned to his care today. You find him pale and weak, with no energy to get out of bed. He also reports pain in his chest.

1. Mr. Frantzis says he is too weak to get up for breakfast. What do you do? _____
_____

2. How do you follow up on the pain in his chest?
_____
_____

3. The nursing assistant assigned to Mr. Frantzis has a runny nose. What should you do? _____
_____

4. Mr. Frantzis calls you "Jennifer" when you enter his room, but that is not your name. How do you respond?
_____
_____

5. You note bleeding from Mr. Frantzis's gums. What care can you provide? _____
_____

CRITICAL THINKING: HODGKIN'S DISEASE

Circle the errors in the following paragraph and write in the correct information.

Joe is a 28-year-old construction worker diagnosed with stage I Hodgkin's disease. He initially went to his physician because of a painful lump in his neck. He is also experiencing high fevers and weight loss. The diagnosis was confirmed in a laboratory test by the presence of Reed-Sternberg cells. He expresses his fears to his nurse, who tells him that Hodgkin's disease is not really cancer, and that it is often curable. Joe takes a leave from work and begins palliative radiation therapy.

SICKLE CELL ANEMIA REVIEW

Fill in the signs and symptoms of sickle cell anemia.

_____

_____

_____

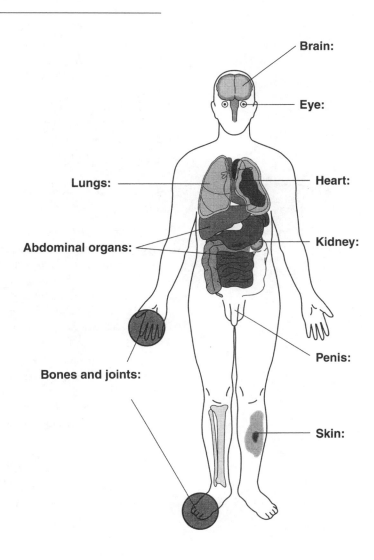

Brain:

Eye:

Lungs:

Heart:

Abdominal organs:

Kidney:

Penis:

Bones and joints:

Skin:

REVIEW QUESTIONS—CONTENT REVIEW

Choose the best answer unless directed otherwise.

1. Which of the following foods will best help provide dietary iron for a patient who has iron-deficiency anemia?
   1. Fresh fruits
   2. Lean red meats
   3. Dairy products
   4. Breads and cereals

2. A 50-year-old African American patient is diagnosed with anemia. Where can the nurse best observe for pallor?
   1. Scalp
   2. Axillae
   3. Chest
   4. Conjunctivae

3. Which of the following is an early sign of anemia?
   1. Palpitations
   2. Glossitis
   3. Pallor
   4. Weight loss

4. For which of the following problems should the nurse monitor in the patient with multiple myeloma?
   1. Uncontrolled bleeding
   2. Respiratory distress
   3. Liver engorgement
   4. Pathological fractures

5. Which of the following interventions can help minimize complications related to hypercalcemia?
   1. Encourage 3 to 4 L of fluid daily.
   2. Have the patient cough and deep breathe every 2 hours.
   3. Place the patient on bedrest.
   4. Apply heat to painful areas.

6. A patient is admitted for a splenectomy. Why is an injection of vitamin K ordered before surgery?
   1. To correct clotting problems
   2. To promote healing
   3. To prevent postoperative infection
   4. To dry secretions

REVIEW QUESTIONS—TEST PREPARATION

Choose the best answer unless directed otherwise.

7. Which of the following conditions places a patient at risk for respiratory complications following splenectomy?
   1. A low platelet count
   2. An incision near the diaphragm
   3. Early ambulation
   4. Early discharge

8. Patients are at risk for overwhelming postsplenectomy infection (OPSI) following splenectomy. Which of the following symptoms alerts the nurse to this possibility?
   1. Bruising around the operative site
   2. Irritability
   3. Pain
   4. Fever

9. A nurse is caring for a patient admitted with gastrointestinal tract bleeding and a hemoglobin level of 6 g/dL. The patient asks the nurse why the low hemoglobin causes shortness of breath. Which response is best?
   1. "Anemia prevents your lungs from absorbing oxygen effectively."
   2. "You do not have enough hemoglobin to carry oxygen to your tissues."
   3. "You don't have enough blood to feed your cells."
   4. "You have lost a lot of blood, and that has damaged your lungs."

10. A 27-year-old African American man is admitted in sickle cell crisis. Which of the following events most likely contributed to the onset of the crisis?
    1. He started a new job last week.
    2. He walked home in a cold rain yesterday.
    3. He had seafood for dinner last night.
    4. He has not exercised for a week.

11. A patient has hand-foot syndrome related to sickle cell anemia. What findings does the nurse expect to see as the patient is examined?
    1. Unequal growth of fingers and toes
    2. Webbing between fingers and toes
    3. Purplish discoloration of hands and feet
    4. Deformities of the wrists and ankles

12. The nurse has taught a patient with thrombocytopenia how to prevent bleeding. Which of the following is the best evidence that the teaching has been effective?
    1. The patient states the importance of avoiding injury.
    2. The patient can list signs and symptoms of bleeding.
    3. The patient uses an electric razor instead of a safety razor.
    4. The patient lists symptoms that should be reported to the doctor.

13. A patient with a history of hemophilia A arrives in the emergency department with a "funny feeling" in his elbow. The patient states that he thinks he is bleeding into the joint. Which response by the nurse is correct?
    1. Palpate the patient's elbow to assess for swelling.
    2. Notify the physician immediately and expect an order for factor VIII.
    3. Prepare the patient for an x-ray examination to determine whether bleeding is occurring.
    4. Apply heat to the elbow and wait for the physician to examine the patient.

14. A patient with a new diagnosis of lymphoma is experiencing fatigue. Which of the following is the best way to assess the fatigue?
    1. Observe the patient's activity level.
    2. Monitor for changes in vital signs.
    3. Monitor hemoglobin and hematocrit values.
    4. Have the patient rate the fatigue on a scale of 0 to 10.

15. A patient diagnosed with lymphoma is being discharged from the hospital. Which of the following statements should the nurse include in the patient teaching?
    1. "It is important to avoid crowds to reduce your risk of infection."
    2. "Taking a walk outside will help reduce your stress level."
    3. "It is important for you to increase your dietary intake of iron."
    4. "Your disease often affects the eyes, so television viewing should be minimized."

16. A patient is having difficulty coping with a new diagnosis of leukemia. Which response by the nurse is most helpful initially?
    1. "Don't worry. You'll be okay."
    2. "The treatments you are receiving will make you feel better very soon."
    3. "Who do you usually go to when you have a problem?"
    4. "Have you made end-of-life decisions?"

17. What discharge teaching is most important to help the patient who has had a splenectomy prevent infection?
    1. Avoid showering for 1 week.
    2. Sleep in a semi-Fowler's position.
    3. Receive a yearly flu vaccine.
    4. Stay on antibiotics for life.

unit SEVEN

Understanding the Respiratory System

CHECKLIST FOR LEARNING SUCCESS

Review of Anatomy and Physiology and Aging Changes	Major Disorders	Nursing Assessment	Diagnostic Tests	Interventions
❑ Lungs and bronchial tree	❑ Epistaxis	❑ Respiratory history	❑ Complete blood count (CBC)	❑ Smoking cessation
❑ Mechanisms of breathing	❑ Upper respiratory infections	❑ Adventitious lung sounds	❑ D-dimer	❑ Interventions for ineffective airway clearance
❑ Acid–base balance	❑ Influenza	❑ Dyspnea	❑ Culture and sensitivity (C&S)	❑ Interventions for impaired gas exchange
❑ Protective mechanisms	❑ Cancer of the larynx	❑ Activity tolerance	❑ TB skin test	
❑ Aging changes	❑ Pneumonia		❑ Oximetry	❑ Positioning
	❑ Tuberculosis (TB)		❑ Capnography	❑ Oxygen therapy
	❑ Restrictive disorders		❑ Arterial blood gases (ABGs)	❑ Nebulized mist treatments
	❑ Chronic obstructive pulmonary disease (COPD)		❑ Chest x-ray	❑ Metered-dose inhalers
	❑ Chronic bronchitis		❑ CT scan	❑ Chest physiotherapy
	❑ Asthma		❑ Ventilation-perfusion scan	❑ Incentive spirometry
	❑ Emphysema		❑ Pulmonary function studies	❑ Chest drainage
	❑ Cystic fibrosis		❑ Pulmonary angiography	❑ Tracheostomy care/suctioning
	❑ Pulmonary embolism		❑ Bronchoscopy	❑ Mechanical ventilation
	❑ Chest trauma			❑ Noninvasive positive pressure ventilation (NIPPV)
	❑ Pneumothorax			
	❑ Respiratory failure			
	❑ Lung cancer			

29

Respiratory System Function, Assessment, and Therapeutic Measures

VOCABULARY

Complete the sentences with the terms provided below.

Adventitious	Barrel	Dyspnea	Thoracentesis	Tracheostomy
Apnea	Crepitus	Excursion	Tidaling	Tracheotomy

1. A patient with a low oxygen saturation may develop _____.

2. _____ may develop if air leaks into tissues from a chest tube site.

3. A _____ may be necessary to reduce distress from severe pleural effusion.

4. The patient with air trapping may develop a _____-shaped chest.

5. The nurse can measure respiratory _____ to check chest expansion.

6. Crackles are an example of a/an _____ sound.

7. A patient who is choking may need an emergency _____.

8. The _____ in the water-seal chamber shows that a chest tube is intact.

9. The absence of respirations is called _____.

10. A patient is taught to remove the inner cannula of a _____ tube every 8 hours for cleaning.

ANATOMY REVIEW

Number the following structures in the order in which air flows through them.

_____ Nose

_____ Trachea

_____ Secondary bronchi

_____ Primary bronchi

_____ Bronchioles

_____ Alveoli

_____ Larynx

_____ Nasopharynx

VENTILATION REVIEW

Number the events of breathing in proper sequence beginning with the medulla.

_____ The medulla generates motor impulses.

_____ The chest cavity is enlarged in all directions.

_____ The diaphragm and external intercostal muscles contract.

_____ Intrapulmonic pressure decreases.

_____ Motor impulses travel along the phrenic and intercostal nerves.

_____ The chest wall expands the parietal pleura, which expands the visceral pleura, which in turn expands the lungs.

_____ Air enters the lungs until intrapulmonic pressure equals atmospheric pressure.

ADVENTITIOUS LUNG SOUNDS

Match the adventitious lung sound to its description.

1. _____ Coarse crackles
2. _____ Fine crackles
3. _____ Wheezes
4. _____ Stridor
5. _____ Pleural friction rub
6. _____ Diminished

1. Velcro® being torn apart
2. Faint lung sounds
3. Leather rubbing together
4. Loud crowing noise
5. Moist bubbling
6. High-pitched violins

CHEST DRAINAGE

Label the three chambers of the chest drainage system and explain the function of each.

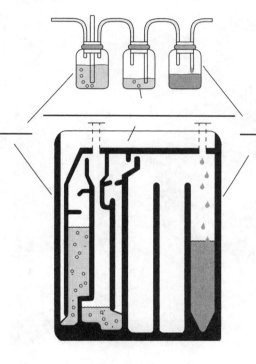

THE RESPIRATORY SYSTEM

Label the parts of the respiratory system.

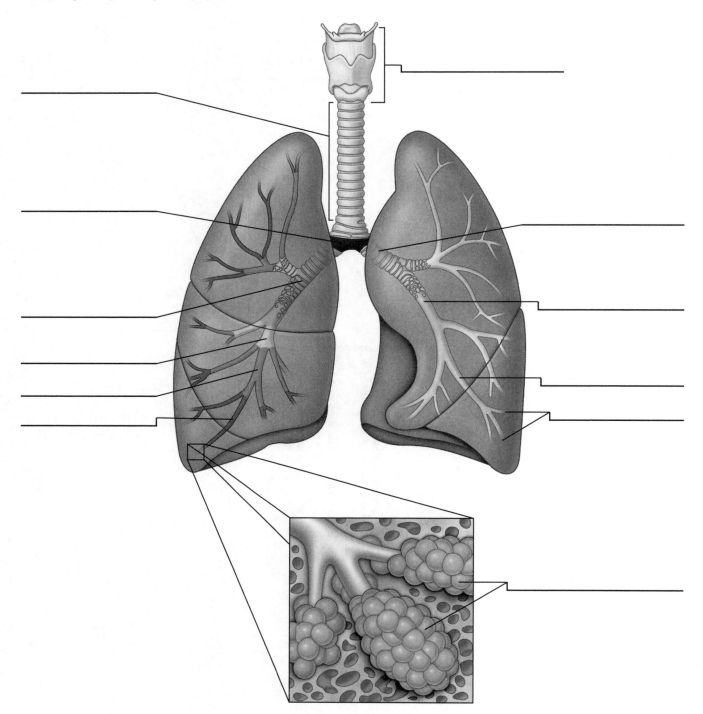

CRITICAL THINKING

Read the following case study and answer the questions.

Bill, a licensed practical nurse (LPN), is collecting admission data on Mr. Howe, who has been admitted for dyspnea and weight loss. While questioning Mr. Howe, Bill learns that he has had progressive weight loss during the past several months and that he has a productive cough. He also reports waking up at night "wringing wet," and his wife has to help him change the bed sheets.

1. What additional questions should Bill ask about Mr. Howe's cough?

   _____

   _____

   _____

2. What disorder is suggested by Mr. Howe's symptoms?

   _____

   _____

   _____

3. What diagnostic tests would you expect to be ordered?

   _____

   _____

   _____

4. Mr. Howe is scheduled for a bronchoscopy. What preprocedure care should Bill provide? Postprocedure?

   _____

   _____

   _____

REVIEW QUESTIONS—CONTENT REVIEW

Choose the best answer unless directed otherwise.

1. Which of the following structures covers the larynx during swallowing?
   1. Hyoid cartilage
   2. Vocal cords
   3. Soft palate
   4. Epiglottis

2. Where are the respiratory centers located in the brain?
   1. Cerebral cortex and cerebellum
   2. Medulla and pons
   3. Hypothalamus and cerebral cortex
   4. Hypothalamus and temporal lobes

3. What is the purpose of the serous fluid between the pleural membranes?
   1. Enhance exchange of gases.
   2. Facilitate coughing.
   3. Destroy pathogens.
   4. Prevent friction.

4. Within the alveoli, surface tension is decreased and inflation is possible because of the presence of which substance?
   1. Tissue fluid
   2. Surfactant
   3. Pulmonary blood
   4. Mucus

5. What is the function of the nasal mucosa?
   1. Assist with gas exchange.
   2. Sweep mucus and pathogens to the trachea.
   3. Warm and moisten the incoming air.
   4. Increase the oxygen content of the air.

6. Deteriorating cilia in the respiratory tract predispose older adults to which of the following problems?
   1. Chronic hypoxia
   2. Pulmonary hypertension
   3. Respiratory infection
   4. Decreased ventilation

7. Which of the following adventitious lung sounds is a violin-like sound?
   1. Crackles
   2. Wheezes
   3. Friction rub
   4. Crepitus

8. The purpose of pursed-lip breathing is to promote which of the following?
   1. Carbon dioxide excretion
   2. Carbon dioxide retention
   3. Oxygen excretion
   4. Oxygen retention

REVIEW QUESTIONS—TEST PREPARATION

Choose the best answer unless directed otherwise.

9. An LPN enters the room of a patient with chronic lung disease. The patient has removed the oxygen cannula, and it is lying on the bed. The patient does not appear to be in any distress. The pulse oximeter shows an oxygen saturation of 79%. Which of the following actions should the nurse take?
   1. Call the registered nurse (RN) STAT.
   2. Put the oxygen cannula back on the patient.
   3. Do a nebulized mist treatment.
   4. No action necessary; this is a normal oxygen saturation.

10. A patient hospitalized with a right-sided pleural effusion calls the nurse and reports feeling short of breath. Which of the following positions should the nurse suggest?
    1. Prone
    2. Supine with head on pillow
    3. Trendelenburg
    4. Side lying with good lung dependent

11. The nurse is caring for a patient with a transtracheal catheter. Which of the following would the LPN expect to be included in the plan of care?
    1. Assist with cleaning the catheter two to three times a day.
    2. Provide supplemental oxygen via mask at all times.
    3. Help remove the catheter at night for sleeping.
    4. Assist to connect the catheter to a humidification source.

12. The wife of a man with cystic fibrosis has been taught how to perform chest physiotherapy. She asks the nurse to explain why this must be done. Which of the following responses is best?
    1. "It helps strengthen chest muscles."
    2. "It humidifies thick respiratory secretions."
    3. "It promotes lung expansion."
    4. "It helps him expectorate secretions."

13. The nurse notes that the suction control chamber on a chest drainage system is bubbling vigorously. Which intervention is appropriate?
    1. Check the system for leaks.
    2. Replace the drainage system with a new one.
    3. Reduce the level of wall suction.
    4. Increase the water level in the suction control chamber.

Nursing Care of Patients With Upper Respiratory Tract Disorders

30

VOCABULARY

Unscramble the letters of the following words to fill in the blanks in the statements below.

hiitsrin   aadihpysg

pixessait   daxueet

laiohnpstry   cayetorlmyng

1. Surgical removal of the voice box is called a _____.

2. A nosebleed is called _____.

3. _____ is the term used to describe drainage or pus.

4. A "nose job" is called _____.

5. Difficulty swallowing is called _____.

6. _____ is the correct term for a runny nose.

CRITICAL THINKING: NASAL SURGERY

Read the following case study and answer the questions.

Mr. Jones had a broken nose as a young man, and now has a deviated nasal septum. He undergoes nasoseptoplasty for a deviated nasal septum.

1. After surgery, you note that Mr. Jones is swallowing repeatedly while he sleeps. What do you do?

   _____

   _____

   _____

2. Before discharge you explain to Mr. Jones that he should not do anything that can increase bleeding, such as sneezing, coughing, or straining to have a bowel movement. He says, "How can I avoid doing those things? It sounds impossible." How do you respond?

   _____

   _____

3. Mr. Jones asks if he can use aspirin for pain. What do you say?

   _____

   _____

CRITICAL THINKING: INFLUENZA

Read the following case study and answer the questions.

Your neighbor calls and describes symptoms of influenza. He is feverish, tired, and has a sore throat and headache. You advise him to go to the urgent care center. The center does a throat culture and determines that the infection is viral. Your neighbor is encouraged to drink fluids and take acetaminophen.

1. Why didn't the health care provider (HCP) order antibiotics? _____

   _____

   _____

2. How will fluids help? _____

   _____

   _____

3. When should the acetaminophen be taken? _____

   _____

   _____

4. Your neighbor's wife develops the same symptoms. Is it necessary to take her to the urgent care center? _____

   _____

   _____

5. Your neighbor's older grandmother was visiting when your neighbor first developed symptoms. She now thinks she has caught the flu, and her chest hurts. She asks what she should do. What should you tell her? _____

   _____

   _____

REVIEW QUESTIONS—CONTENT REVIEW

Choose the best answer unless directed otherwise.

1. When evaluating the effectiveness of nursing interventions for sinusitis pain, which data does the nurse collect?
   1. White blood cell (WBC) count
   2. Amount and color of sinus drainage
   3. Capillary refill
   4. Pain level on a 0 to 10 scale

2. Which of the following communication methods is inappropriate for a patient following laryngectomy surgery?
   1. Placing a finger over the stoma
   2. Using a special valve that diverts air into the esophagus
   3. Using a picture board
   4. Learning esophageal speech

3. Why are narcotics given in low doses for pain to the patient who has had a laryngectomy?
   1. They depress the respiratory rate and cough reflex.
   2. They increase respiratory tract secretions.
   3. They have a tendency to cause stomal edema.
   4. They can cause addiction.

4. A 58-year-old man is diagnosed with cancer of the larynx. Which of the following are early symptoms of this cancer?
   1. Anemia and fatigue
   2. Crackles and stridor
   3. A noticeable lump in the neck
   4. Dysphagia or hoarseness

5. A patient visits a nurse practitioner (NP) after having a cold for a week; the patient is now experiencing a severe headache and fever. The NP diagnoses a sinus infection. Which of the following additional symptoms is the patient likely to exhibit?
   1. Facial tenderness
   2. Chest pain
   3. Photophobia
   4. Ear drainage

REVIEW QUESTIONS—TEST PREPARATION

Choose the best answer unless directed otherwise.

6. In addition to antibiotics, which of the following recommendations can the nurse make to increase comfort for a patient experiencing sinusitis? **Select all that apply.**
   1. Coughing and deep breathing
   2. Sinus irrigation
   3. Hot moist packs
   4. Room humidifier
   5. Percussion and postural drainage
   6. Semi-Fowler's position

7. Place the following four nursing actions for a patient who has just had a laryngectomy in correct order of priority.
   1. Assist with ambulation.
   2. Set up a visit from a well-adjusted patient who has had a laryngectomy.
   3. Maintain a patent airway.
   4. Control postoperative pain.

8. The nurse teaches a patient how to live with a new tracheostomy. Which of the following instructions is appropriate?
   1. "Never suction your tracheostomy; you might damage your trachea."
   2. "You should not feel bad about the tracheostomy—you should feel lucky to be alive."
   3. "Be sure to protect your tracheostomy from pollutants such as powders or hair."
   4. "Your tracheostomy will be cleaned each time you visit your doctor."

9. A 17-year-old student enters the emergency department with a nosebleed that won't stop. Which of the following positions should the nurse assist the patient to assume?
   1. Lying down with feet elevated
   2. Sitting up with neck extended
   3. Lying down with a small pillow under the head
   4. Sitting up leaning slightly forward

10. The physician orders local application of phenylephrine solution to treat a nosebleed. The patient asks how this will help. Which of the following responses by the nurse is best?
    1. "It will raise your blood pressure, which is necessary because of blood loss."
    2. "It will dilate your bronchioles and make your breathing easier."
    3. "It will help your blood to clot to reduce bleeding."
    4. "It will constrict your vessels and slow down the bleeding."

11. A nurse is providing community education related to swine flu. Which of the following statements by a participant indicates that teaching has been effective?
    1. "I've eliminated all pork from my diet."
    2. "Swine flu can only be transmitted by pigs."
    3. "Symptoms of swine flu are similar to other types of flu."
    4. "There is a new medication just for swine flu treatment."

31

Nursing Care of Patients With Lower Respiratory Tract Disorders

VOCABULARY

Complete the crossword puzzle.

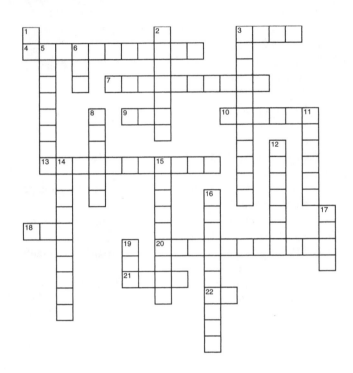

Across

3. Acronym for a syndrome that is also called "white lung"
4. Chest collapses during inspiration with this type of respiration
7. Bloody sputum
9. Abbreviation for inhaler
10. Respiratory membrane secretion
13. Incision into the chest
18. Abbreviation for inhaled nebulized medication
20. Treatment for repeat pneumothorax
21. Blister on lung
22. Abbreviation for tuberculosis

Down

1. Abbreviation for "front to back" when referring to the chest
2. Term used to describe hormones produced by tumors
3. Medication that relieves coughing
5. Treatment in addition to standard therapy
6. Abbreviation for laboratory tests done to measure respiratory status
8. Unable to react, as in skin testing
11. Continuous asthma is called _____ asthmaticus.
12. Drainage on infected tonsils
14. Blood in the chest
15. Rapid respirations
16. Firm raised area in positive tuberculosis skin test
17. Smoking is a _____ factor for cancer
19. Abbreviation for short of breath

RESPIRATORY MEDICATIONS

Match the medication with its action.

1. _____ Prednisone

2. _____ Albuterol (Ventolin)

3. _____ Tiotropium (Spiriva)

4. _____ Cromolyn sodium (Intal)

5. _____ Guaifenesin (Humibid)

6. _____ Zafirlukast (Accolate)

7. _____ Codeine

1. Expectorant

2. Potent anti-inflammatory

3. Leukotriene inhibitor (reduces inflammation in asthma)

4. Short-acting beta-agonist bronchodilator

5. Anticholinergic bronchodilator

6. Mast cell stabilizer to prevent asthma symptoms

7. Antitussive

CRITICAL THINKING

Read the following case study and answer the questions.

Edith is a 56-year-old homemaker admitted to the hospital with emphysema and acute dyspnea. She is a smoker with a 48-pack-year history.

1. What data do you collect for Edith's admission database?

2. What does a 48-pack-year history mean?

3. Explain the pathophysiology involved in emphysema. How does the disease cause dyspnea?

4. What do you expect Edith's lungs to sound like when you auscultate?

5. Why is it important for Edith to receive no more than 2 L of oxygen per minute, unless she is closely monitored?

6. Why might Edith be at risk for pneumothorax?

7. What position will help Edith's shortness of breath? Why?

8. How can you encourage Edith to stop smoking?

_____

_____

_____

REVIEW QUESTIONS—CONTENT REVIEW

Choose the best answer unless directed otherwise.

1. A patient is treated with intravenous (IV) methylpred-
   nisolone (Solu-Medrol) for emphysema. What is the
   purpose of corticosteroid treatment in lung disease?
   1. Dry secretions.
   2. Treat the infection that causes an exacerbation.
   3. Improve the oxygen-carrying capacity of hemoglobin.
   4. Reduce airway inflammation.

2. How many liters per minute of oxygen should be administered to the patient with emphysema?
   1. 2 L/min
   2. 6 L/min
   3. 10 L/min
   4. 95 L/min

3. Which of the following medications can be used to
   quickly reduce shortness of breath in a crisis situation
   for a patient with end-stage respiratory disease?
   1. Oral cortisone
   2. Intramuscular meperidine (Demerol)
   3. IV morphine
   4. IV propranolol (Inderal)

4. Which of the following risk factors presents the greatest
   threat for respiratory disease?
   1. Smoking
   2. High-fat diet
   3. Exposure to radiation
   4. Alcohol consumption

REVIEW QUESTIONS—TEST PREPARATION

Choose the best answer unless directed otherwise.

5. A 72-year-old retired chemist has left lower lobe pneumonia. The nurse checks the patient's oxygen saturation
   and the result is 86%. Which of the following actions by
   the nurse is best?
   1. Contact the registered nurse (RN) or physician for an
      order for oxygen.
   2. No action necessary; this is a normal SpO_2.
   3. Call the respiratory therapist STAT for assistance.
   4. Walk the patient in the hall and recheck the O_2
      saturation.

6. The nurse is caring for a patient who is scheduled for a
   bronchoscopy. Which of the following would be included in preprocedure teaching?
   1. "The physician will place a small tube through your
      nose or mouth and into the bronchi to look at your
      airways."
   2. "You will breathe a radioactive substance that will
      show diseased areas in your lungs."
   3. "You will need to drink a thick white liquid, which
      will be opaque on the x-rays."
   4. "A dye will be injected to help visualize the struc-
      tures of the bronchioles. Do you have any allergies?"

7. A patient is returned to the room after a bronchoscopy.
   Which of the following actions should the nurse
   take first?
   1. Order a meal because the patient has been nil per os
      (NPO) for 8 hours.
   2. Encourage fluids to flush dye from the patient's
      system.
   3. Monitor the patient for return to consciousness.
   4. Check for a gag reflex before allowing the patient
      to drink.

8. A patient asks how to avoid lung cancer. Which of the
   following should the nurse include in the patient teaching? **Select all that apply.**
   1. Live in a cold climate.
   2. Stop smoking.
   3. Avoid exposure to passive smoke.
   4. Avoid air pollution.
   5. Avoid crowded living conditions.
   6. Consume a diet high in fruits and vegetables.

9. A patient with a new diagnosis of small cell lung cancer
   decides to have radiation therapy. Which of the following expectations of this treatment is most appropriate?
   1. Complete cure of the cancer
   2. Increased comfort
   3. Prevention of the need for oxygen
   4. Prevention of cancer spread

10. A newly diagnosed patient asks the nurse to explain asthma. Which of the following explanations by the nurse is correct?
    1. "Your airways are inflamed and spastic."
    2. "You have fluid in your lungs that is causing shortness of breath."
    3. "Your airways are stretched and nonfunctional."
    4. "You have a low-grade infection that keeps your bronchial tree irritated."

11. Which of the following is the best explanation of emphysema for a newly diagnosed patient?
    1. "You have inflamed bronchioles, which causes a lot of secretions."
    2. "The blood vessels that supply your lungs are damaged, so you can't absorb oxygen."
    3. "Your lungs have lost some of their elasticity, and air gets trapped."
    4. "You have large dilated sacs of sputum in your lungs."

12. How can the nurse help monitor effectiveness of therapy for the patient with a pneumothorax and a chest drainage system?
    1. Palpate for crepitus.
    2. Auscultate lung sounds.
    3. Document color and amount of sputum.
    4. Monitor suction level.

unit EIGHT

Understanding the Gastrointestinal, Hepatic, and Pancreatic Systems

CHECKLIST FOR LEARNING SUCCESS

Review of Anatomy and Physiology and Aging Changes
- ❑ Gastrointestinal (GI):
- ❑ Oral cavity/pharynx
- ❑ Esophagus
- ❑ Stomach
- ❑ Small intestine
- ❑ Large intestine
- ❑ Aging
- ❑ Liver structure and function
- ❑ Gallbladder structure and function
- ❑ Pancreas structure and function
- ❑ Aging changes

Major Disorders
- ❑ Oral disorders
- ❑ Nausea/vomiting
- ❑ Eating disorders
- ❑ Oral/esophageal cancer
- ❑ Gastroesophageal reflux disease (GERD)
- ❑ Gastritis
- ❑ Peptic ulcer disease
- ❑ Gastric bleeding
- ❑ Gastric cancer
- ❑ Constipation/diarrhea
- ❑ Appendicitis
- ❑ Peritonitis
- ❑ Diverticulosis
- ❑ Inflammatory bowel disease
- ❑ Absorption disorders
- ❑ Intestinal obstructions
- ❑ Lower gastrointestinal (GI) bleeding
- ❑ Colon cancer
- ❑ Hepatitis
- ❑ Liver failure
- ❑ Pancreatitis
- ❑ Cholecystitis
- ❑ Cholelithiasis
- ❑ Cancer

Nursing Assessment
- ❑ Nursing data collection
- ❑ Medical history
- ❑ Physical examination
- ❑ Pain
- ❑ Alcohol use history
- ❑ Medication history
- ❑ GI signs and symptoms
- ❑ Skin
- ❑ Abdomen
- ❑ Mental status

Diagnostic Tests
- ❑ Laboratory tests
- ❑ Flat plate of abdomen
- ❑ Upper GI series
- ❑ Lower GI series
- ❑ Esophagogastroduodenoscopy (EGD)
- ❑ Colonoscopy
- ❑ Gastric analysis
- ❑ Stool studies
- ❑ Immunoglobulin G antibody test
- ❑ Alanine transaminase, Aspartate transaminase
- ❑ Albumin
- ❑ Amylase
- ❑ Ammonia
- ❑ Bilirubin
- ❑ Prothrombin time
- ❑ Occult blood
- ❑ Upper GI, lower GI series
- ❑ Cholecystogram
- ❑ Liver scan
- ❑ Endoscopic retrograde cholangiopancreatography
- ❑ Liver biopsy

Interventions
- ❑ GI intubation
- ❑ Tube feedings
- ❑ Parenteral nutrition
- ❑ GI decompression
- ❑ Gastric surgeries/complications
- ❑ Nursing care after gastric surgery
- ❑ Ostomy management
- ❑ Transjugular intrahepatic portosystemic shunt
- ❑ Tamponade
- ❑ Transplant
- ❑ Cholecystectomy
- ❑ Nutrition
- ❑ Pain control

Common Medications
- ❑ Antacids
- ❑ Antidiarrheals
- ❑ Antiemetics
- ❑ Bulk-forming agents
- ❑ H_2 receptor antagonists
- ❑ Laxatives
- ❑ Proton pump inhibitors
- ❑ Stool softeners
- ❑ Vitamin B_{12}
- ❑ Diuretics
- ❑ Analgesics
- ❑ Histamine antagonists
- ❑ Lactulose
- ❑ Neomycin

32

Gastrointestinal, Hepatobiliary, and Pancreatic Systems Function, Assessment, and Therapeutic Measures

FUNCTIONS OF THE GASTROINTESTINAL SYSTEM

Fill in the blanks with the appropriate parts of the gastrointestinal (GI) system.

1. The _____ sphincter prevents backup of stomach contents into the esophagus.
2. The _____ valve prevents backup of fecal material from the large intestine into the small intestine.
3. The _____ sphincter prevents backup of duodenal contents into the stomach.
4. The absorption of most of the end products of digestion occurs in the _____ intestine.
5. The digestion of protein begins in the _____.
6. Water and the vitamins produced by the normal flora are absorbed in the _____ intestine.
7. The _____ intestine is the site of action of bile and pancreatic enzymes.
8. The passageway for food into the stomach from the mouth is the _____.
9. Voluntary control of defecation is provided by the _____ sphincter.
10. The watery secretion that permits taste and swallowing is produced by the _____ glands.
11. The process of mechanical digestion is accomplished by the _____ and _____ in the mouth.
12. The structures in the small intestine that contain capillaries and lacteals for absorption are the _____.
13. The part of the colon that contracts in the defecation reflex is the _____.
14. The digestive function of the liver is the production of _____ by the hepatocytes.

STRUCTURES OF THE GASTROINTESTINAL SYSTEM

Label the following structures.

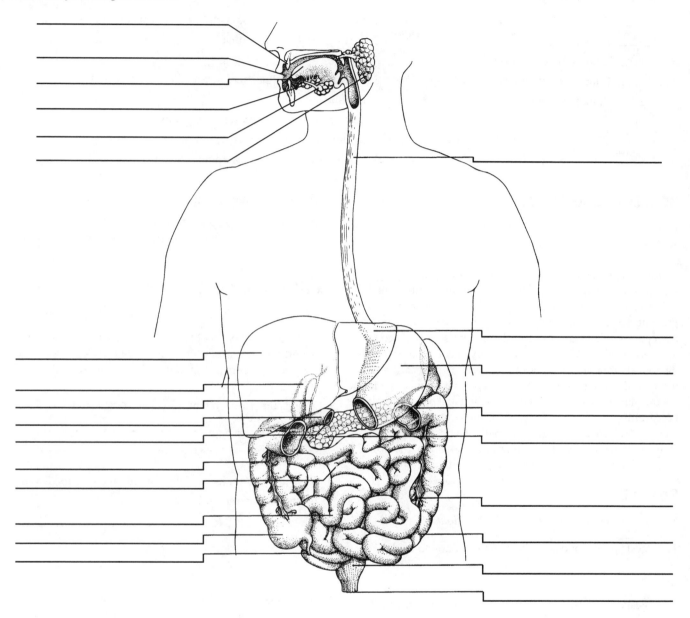

VOCABULARY

Unscramble the letters to identify the word described by the definition.

1. Flexible or rigid device consisting of a tube and optical system for observing the inside of a hollow organ or cavity. _____ donscepeo

2. Gurgling and clicking heard over the abdomen caused by air and fluid movement from peristaltic action normally occurring every 5 to 15 seconds at a rate of 5 to 35 per minute. _____ wlebo onudss

3. Examination of the upper portion of the rectum with an endoscope. _____ locnooscypo

4. Feeding via a tube placed in the stomach. _____ gvaaeg

5. Immovable accumulation of feces in the bowels. _____ mipcaitno

6. Resin obtained from trees to test for occult blood in feces. _____ gaiuca

7. Device consisting of a fluorescent screen that makes the shadows of objects interposed between the tube and the screen visible. _____ ulfroocspeo

8. Fatty stools. _____ estaotrhrae

9. A test performed to measure secretions of hydrochloric acid and pepsin in the stomach. _____ stgairc naayliss

10. Examination of the stomach and abdominal cavity by use of an endoscope. _____ stgarsopcoy

LABORATORY TESTS

Match the test with its definition.

1. _____ Stool for lipids
2. _____ Stool cultures
3. _____ Stool for occult blood
4. _____ Carcinoembryonic antigen (CEA)
5. _____ Stool for ova and parasites

1. Levels may indicate colorectal or other cancer.
2. Testing stool for blood that is not visible to the eye
3. Testing stool for intestinal infections caused by parasites
4. Testing stool for the presence of pathogenic organisms in the GI tract
5. Testing stool for excessive amounts of fat

BOWEL PREPARATION

Circle the eight errors in the following paragraph, and insert the correct information.

A stomach preparation is required for several procedures that visualize the lower bowel. This preparation is important for effective test results. An incomplete bowel preparation may prevent the test from being done or cause the need for it to be repeated. This can result in the patient's early discharge and cost savings. The patient usually receives a soft diet 24 hours before the test. A bowel preparation medication (liquid or pill) may be given. A cool tap-water enema or Fleet enema may be given once. Older or debilitated patients should be carefully assessed during the administration of multiple enemas, which can fatigue the patient and increase electrolytes. In patients with bleeding or constipation, the bowel preparation may not be ordered by the health care provider.

PANCREAS

State the pancreatic enzyme with its function.

1. Digests polypeptides to short chains of amino acids.

   _____

2. Digests emulsified fats to fatty acids and glycerol.

   _____

3. Digests starch to maltose.

   _____

LIVER

Fill in the blanks with the appropriate words.

1. Liver or gallbladder disease may cause pale or _____ colored stools.
2. Liver disease may cause _____ disorders.
3. A liver scan records the amount of _____ material taken up by the liver to form a composite "picture" of the liver.

4. After a liver biopsy, the patient lies on the right side for the first _____ hours.
5. After a liver biopsy, nursing care focuses on monitoring for _____.

CRITICAL THINKING

Read the following case study and answer the questions.

Mrs. Davis is a 41-year-old schoolteacher who is admitted to your unit with recurrent lung cancer. She is debilitated and her physician orders parenteral nutrition to be started.

1. Why is the parenteral nutrition rate started slowly at first?

   _____

   _____

2. Why are serum glucose levels monitored on Mrs. Davis during parenteral nutrition administration?

   _____

   _____

   _____

3. In what types of veins may parenteral nutrition be administered with (a) dextrose of 12% or less; (b) dextrose greater than 12%? _____

   _____

4. Why is it necessary to use an infusion control pump for parenteral nutrition? _____

   _____

5. The parenteral nutrition is behind schedule. What action should the nurse take? _____

   _____

6. When parenteral nutrition is discontinued, why might the infusion be slowly weaned off? _____

_____

_____

7. When parenteral nutrition is ordered to be stopped, why should the patient be fed first, if it is not contraindicated? _____

_____

8. Identify one nursing diagnosis and outcome with interventions for the patient on parenteral nutrition.

Nursing Diagnosis _____

_____

Patient Outcome _____

_____

Interventions _____

_____

_____

REVIEW QUESTIONS—CONTENT REVIEW

Choose the best answer unless directed otherwise.

1. Which of the following structures are connected by the ileocecal valve?
   1. Duodenum to the stomach
   2. Colon to the small intestine
   3. Stomach to the esophagus
   4. Ileum to the jejunum

2. Mechanical digestion in the stomach is accomplished by which of the following structures?
   1. Mucosa
   2. Smooth muscle layers
   3. Striated muscle layers
   4. Gastric glands

3. Gastric juice contributes to the digestion of which of the following types of nutrients?
   1. Proteins
   2. Fats
   3. Starch

4. The enzymes of the small intestine contribute to the digestion of which of the following types of nutrients?
   1. Proteins
   2. Fats
   3. Disaccharides

5. Which of the following structures carries bile and pancreatic juices to the duodenum?
   1. Pancreatic duct
   2. Cystic duct
   3. Hepatic duct
   4. Common bile duct

6. Which of the following is a function of the liver?
   1. Synthesis of plasma proteins
   2. Elimination of carbohydrates
   3. Concentration of bile
   4. Secretion of cholecystokinin

7. Which of the following diagnostic procedures on stool specimens must the nurse collect using sterile technique?
   1. Stool for ova and parasites
   2. Stool for occult blood
   3. Stool culture
   4. Stool for lipids

8. Which of the following colors would the nurse recognize as an expected finding for the patient's stools immediately after a barium swallow?
   1. Brown
   2. Black
   3. White
   4. Green

9. Which of the following does the nurse understand is the primary reason a patient is non per os (NPO) until the gag reflex returns after an esophagogastroduodenoscopy (EGD) procedure?
   1. To rest the vocal cords
   2. To prevent aspiration
   3. To keep the throat dry
   4. To prevent vomiting

10. Which of the following positions would the nurse be correct in using for nasogastric (NG) tube insertion?
    1. Trendelenburg's
    2. Prone
    3. Sims'
    4. High-Fowler's

REVIEW QUESTIONS—TEST PREPARATION

Choose the best answer unless directed otherwise.

11. Bowel sounds heard as soft clicks and gurgles at a rate of 4 per minute would be documented by the nurse as which of the following types of findings?
    1. Absent
    2. Hyperactive
    3. Hypoactive
    4. Normal

12. Which of the following diagnostic procedures requires that a patient be NPO? **Select all that apply.**
    1. Upper GI series (barium swallow)
    2. Flat plate of the abdomen
    3. EGD
    4. Computed tomography (CT) scan
    5. Endoscopic retrograde cholangiopancreatography (ERCP)

13. Which of the following nursing diagnoses would be most appropriate to include in the patient's plan of care after a barium swallow? **Select all that apply.**
    1. Risk for Constipation
    2. Risk for Diarrhea
    3. Risk for Pain
    4. Imbalanced Nutrition: More Than Body Requirements
    5. Deficient Knowledge

14. A patient who has an NG tube and an intravenous (IV) line states, "I'm so embarrassed to have my family here I have tubes coming out of me everywhere." Which of the following would be an appropriate nursing diagnosis?
    1. Fear
    2. Defensive Coping
    3. Disturbed Body Image
    4. Anxiety

15. In preparing a patient who is to have an NG tube inserted, which of the following statements would the nurse include in the patient teaching?
    1. "This procedure often makes you cough."
    2. "You can help by swallowing or drinking liquids during the procedure."
    3. "It is very important that you hold your breath when I tell you to do so."
    4. "When instructed, I want you to exhale as quickly and forcefully as you can."

Nursing Care of Patients With Upper Gastrointestinal Disorders

33

VOCABULARY

Unscramble the letters to identify a word described by the definition.

1. Most common cause of peptic ulcers; its discovery has revolutionized treatment and cure of most peptic ulcers. _____ lehicbocatre ypoilr
2. Loss of appetite _____ noraxeai
3. Inflammation of the stomach _____ sagrtisti
4. Small, white, painful ulcers that appear on the inner cheeks, lips, gums, tongue, palate, and pharynx _____ hpatouhs tsoamtisti
5. Recurrent episodes of binge eating and self-induced vomiting _____ lubiami ernvsoa
6. Rapid entry of food into the jejunum causing dizziness, tachycardia, fainting, sweating, nausea, diarrhea, and abdominal cramping _____ umdpnig nysdomre
7. Surgical removal of the stomach _____ gtrasetcmyo
8. 20% to 30% over average weight for age, sex, and height _____ boesiyt
9. Condition in which the stomach may protrude above the diaphragm _____ ihaatl erhian
10. Following surgical removal of part of the stomach, reanastomosis of the remaining portion to the proximal jejunum _____ satgorjujeonsotym

---

GASTRITIS

Match the description with the type of gastritis associated with it.

1. _____ Heartburn or indigestion
2. _____ Autoimmune gastritis
3. _____ Often caused by overeating
4. _____ Associated with the bacteria *Helicobacter pylori*
5. _____ Associated with difficulty in absorbing vitamin B_{12}
6. _____ Can lead to peritonitis
7. _____ Can be treated with antibiotics
8. _____ Treatment includes a bland diet

1. Acute gastritis
2. Chronic gastritis type A
3. Chronic gastritis type B

PEPTIC ULCER DISEASE

Circle the seven errors in the following paragraph and write the correct information.

Most peptic ulcers are caused by stress. Peptic ulcers are commonly found in the sigmoid colon. Symptoms of peptic ulcers include burning and a gnawing pain in the chest. With a duodenal ulcer, there is pain and discomfort with a full stomach, which may be relieved by avoiding food. Peptic ulcers cannot be cured. Medication treatment for most peptic ulcers should include anticoagulants as indicated.

GASTRECTOMY

Label the structures as they appear following various types of gastric surgery.

CRITICAL THINKING

Read the following case study and answer the questions.

Mrs. Sheffield has just returned from surgery. She had a gastroduodenostomy (Billroth I) procedure. She has a nasogastric (NG) tube, a 1000-mL intravenous (IV) of lactated Ringer's solution infusing at 100 mL/hr, and a Foley catheter. She is nil per os (NPO). Her vital signs are stable: blood pressure 118/90 mm Hg, pulse 80 beats per minute, respirations 16 per minute, and temperature 98°F (36.6°C). Her abdominal dressing is clean, dry, and intact. She is drowsy but easily aroused. After getting Mrs. Sheffield settled in bed, the nurse connects her NG tube to intermittent low-wall suction as ordered by her health care provider (HCP) and adds another blanket to warm her. Mrs. Sheffield requests something for pain. The nurse administers morphine 5 mg intramuscularly

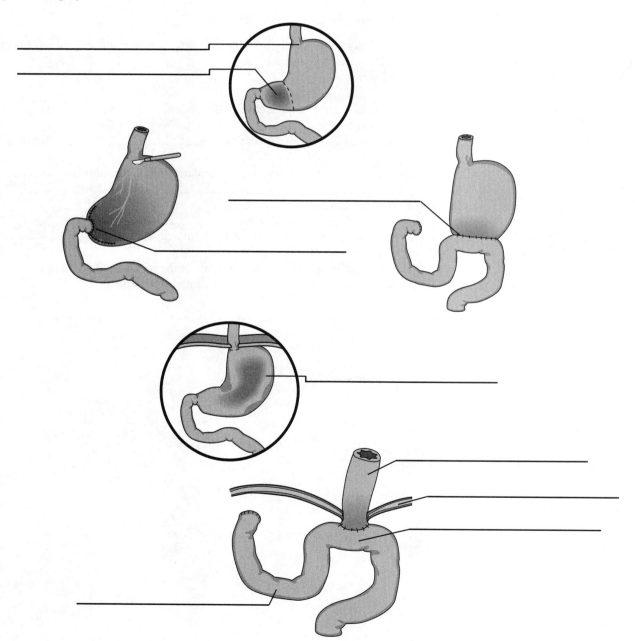

and allows her to rest. An hour later, the nursing assistant tells the nurse that Mrs. Sheffield is vomiting bright red blood. The nurse goes to her room and finds her lying on her side propped up on one arm vomiting into an emesis basin. Her NG suction catheter contains 250 mL of bright red drainage. Her dressing remains clean and dry. She is diaphoretic and reporting nausea.

1. What should be the nurse's first response?

   _____

   _____

2. What is the nurse's next action?

   _____

   _____

3. Vital signs are now blood pressure 86/60 mm Hg, pulse 96 beats per minute, respirations 24 per minute, and temperature 97.6°F (36.4°C). What is the nurse's assessment of the new data, and what is the nurse's next step?

   _____

   _____

4. As the nurse lightly palpates Mrs. Sheffield's abdomen, it feels slightly distended, and the nurse suspects that she may be bleeding into her peritoneum. What is the nurse's next step? _____

   _____

5. What should the nurse tell the HCP?

   _____

   _____

6. The HCP orders a stat hematocrit and hemoglobin, electrolytes, and oxygen at 2 L/min via nasal cannula. The HCP also tells the nurse to get Mrs. Sheffield ready to return to surgery. What is the nurse's priority nursing action?

   _____

   _____

REVIEW QUESTIONS—CONTENT REVIEW

Choose the best answer unless directed otherwise.

1. Which of the following surgical procedures is the most likely treatment for a patient with gastric cancer?
   1. Gastroplasty
   2. Gastrorrhaphy
   3. Gastric stapling
   4. Gastrectomy

2. Which of the following does the nurse understand is a sign or symptom of oral cancer?
   1. Painless ulcer
   2. White painful ulcers
   3. Feeling of fullness
   4. Heartburn

3. Which of the following procedures does the nurse understand is done palliatively for the dysphagia that occurs in inoperable esophageal cancer?
   1. Gastrectomy
   2. Esophageal dilation
   3. Radical neck dissection
   4. Modified neck dissection

REVIEW QUESTIONS—TEST PREPARATION

Choose the best answer unless directed otherwise.

4. A patient has a duodenal peptic ulcer and is taking cimetidine (Tagamet). Which of the following side effects related to cimetidine should be included in the teaching plan?
   1. Confusion
   2. Hypertension
   3. Blurred vision
   4. Dry mouth

5. A patient is admitted with chronic gastritis type B. Which of the following signs and symptoms is the nurse likely to find on assessment?
   1. Anorexia
   2. Dysphagia
   3. Diarrhea
   4. Feeling of fullness

6. An asymptomatic patient is admitted with gastric bleeding. For which of the following signs or symptoms of severe gastric bleeding should the nurse monitor? **Select all that apply.**
   1. Hypertension
   2. Diaphoresis
   3. Bounding pulse
   4. Hypotension
   5. Confusion

7. A patient had a gastrectomy 2 months ago. The patient comes to the clinic for treatment for greasy stools and frequent bowel movements. After the patient's surgical recovery and current eating habits are assessed, which of the following types of diet would be most appropriate for the nurse to teach the patient to use?
   1. Bland diet
   2. High-carbohydrate diet
   3. Low-fat diet
   4. Pureed diet

8. A patient visits her HCP and reports that she is very unhappy with her weight, which is 310 lb on her 5-foot 7-inch frame. When planning her care, the nurse knows that the initial treatment for obesity includes which of the following?
   1. Gastroplasty
   2. Billroth I procedure
   3. Billroth II procedure
   4. Diet management

9. A patient has been diagnosed with a hiatal hernia. The patient has heartburn and occasional regurgitation. Which of the following interventions should the nurse teach the patient to reduce the symptoms?
   1. Eat small, frequent meals.
   2. Recline for 1 hour after meals.
   3. Sleep flat without a pillow.
   4. Eat a bedtime snack.

10. A patient is having an acute episode of gastric bleeding. The HCP orders an IV of 1000 mL of 0.9% normal saline, a complete blood cell (CBC) count, a nasogastric tube to low-wall suction, and oxygen by nasal cannula. Which of the following orders should the nurse perform first?
    1. Administer the IV of 1000 mL of 0.9% normal saline.
    2. Draw the blood for the CBC cell.
    3. Insert the NG tube.
    4. Apply oxygen by nasal cannula.

11. A patient is taught preventive measure for gastroesophageal reflux disease. Which of the following patient statements indicates that teaching has been effective?
    1. "I need to eat large meals."
    2. "I will sleep without pillows."
    3. "I need to lie down for 2 hours after each meal."
    4. "I will identify foods that cause discomfort."

12. The nurse is caring for a patient who recently returned from surgery after fundoplication. Which of the following symptoms is essential to report to the physician?
    1. Nausea
    2. Pain rated as 4 out of 10
    3. Dysphagia
    4. Thirst

Nursing Care of Patients With Lower Gastrointestinal Disorders

34

VOCABULARY

Match the vocabulary word to the correct definition.

1. _____ Appendicitis
2. _____ Colectomy
3. _____ Colitis
4. _____ Colostomy
5. _____ Diverticulosis
6. _____ Fistula
7. _____ Hernia
8. _____ Ileostomy
9. _____ Intussusception
10. _____ Melena
11. _____ Peritonitis
12. _____ Volvulus

1. Outpouchings in colon
2. Inflammation of colon
3. Telescoping of the bowel
4. Tunnel connection between bowel and another organ
5. Blood in stool
6. Twisting of bowel
7. Inflammation or infection of peritoneum
8. Bulging of abdominal contents through abdominal wall
9. Diversion of small bowel through abdominal wall
10. Removal of large bowel
11. Diversion of large bowel through abdominal wall
12. Inflamed appendix

OSTOMIES

Circle the four errors in each of the following paragraphs and insert the correct information.

1. Michelle Braun is a 16-year-old with ulcerative colitis. She is taking cortisone. She is on a high-residue diet. She has just been admitted to the hospital for a colectomy and elective loop ostomy. The nurse monitors her intake and output (I&O), daily weights, and electrolytes. The nurse also monitors for signs of inflammation in her joints, skin, and other parts of her body. The nurse teaches her to restrict fluids following surgery to limit the number of stools she has daily.

   _____

   _____

2. James Key is a 46-year-old with a new sigmoid colostomy. Following surgery the nurse monitors his stoma every shift for 3 days to ensure that it remains gray and moist. The nurse explains that the stool will be semiformed and that he will have to irrigate his ostomy every 1 to 2 days to have bowel movements. The nurse contacts the dietitian to provide a list of the high-fiber foods that he should eat.

CRITICAL THINKING

Read the following case study and answer the questions.

Mrs. Millie Hendricks is a 90-year-old resident in a nursing home. Mrs. Hendricks has a history of severe osteoarthritis, and she has no teeth or dentures, but otherwise she is quite healthy. She normally has a bowel movement every other day but has occasional constipation, which she takes care of herself by requesting a dose of milk of magnesia. Today when the nurse takes Mrs. Hendricks's medications to her, she says, "I think I need a second dose of that milk of magnesia; my bowels haven't moved in 3 days." The nurse looks at the medication administration record and finds as needed (prn) orders for milk of magnesia, psyllium (Metamucil), senna (Senokot), or a tap water enema.

1. What should the nurse do before administering more medication?

_____

_____

_____

_____

2. What factors most likely led to Mrs. Hendricks's constipation?

_____

_____

_____

_____

3. What will happen if Mrs. Hendricks's bowels do not move today?

_____

_____

_____

_____

4. What nondrug interventions will help Mrs. Hendricks move her bowels?

_____

_____

_____

_____

5. After Mrs. Hendricks's bowels have moved, what measures can be instituted to prevent constipation next time?

_____

_____

_____

_____

REVIEW QUESTIONS—CONTENT REVIEW

Choose the best answer unless directed otherwise.

1. What differentiates diverticulitis from diverticulosis? **Select all that apply.**
   1. Presence of weakness in bowel wall
   2. Presence of outpouchings on bowel mucous membrane
   3. Presence of inflammation and infection
   4. Lack of symptoms
   5. Involves the large intestine.

2. A pattern of alternating constipation and diarrhea is most characteristic of which of the following gastrointestinal (GI) tract disorders?
   1. Crohn's disease
   2. Ulcerative colitis
   3. Irritable bowel syndrome (IBS)
   4. Large bowel obstruction

3. Which of the following drugs would the nurse expect to be prescribed for a woman with IBS and constipation?
   1. Amitriptyline (Elavil)
   2. Dicyclomine (Bentyl)
   3. Paroxetine HCl (Paxil)
   4. Hyoscyamine (Levbid)

REVIEW QUESTIONS—TEST PREPARATION

Choose the best answer unless directed otherwise.

4. A patient who has ulcerative colitis is taken to the emergency department with severe rectal bleeding. Which of the following is the best option for maintaining nutritional status for this patient with ulcerative colitis who must be nil per os (NPO) for an extended period of time?
   1. Nasogastric (NG) tube feedings
   2. Percutaneous endoscopic gastrostomy (PEG) tube feedings
   3. Parenteral nutrition (PN)
   4. Intravenous (IV) 5% dextrose and water

5. A patient is diagnosed with acute diverticulitis. Which of the following may have placed the patient at risk for developing diverticulitis?
   1. Eating a low-fiber diet
   2. Chronic diarrhea
   3. History of nonsteroidal anti-inflammatory drug (NSAID) use
   4. Family history of colon cancer

6. Which of the following foods might a patient with diverticulitis be instructed to avoid?
   1. Peanuts and raspberries
   2. Apples and pears
   3. Red meat and dairy products
   4. Bran and whole grains

7. Which of the following nursing diagnoses is most appropriate to include in the plan of care for a patient with symptoms of a bowel obstruction?
   1. *Risk for Impaired Swallowing* related to NPO status
   2. *Risk for Urinary Retention* related to fluid volume depletion
   3. *Risk for Deficient Fluid Volume* related to nausea and vomiting
   4. *Risk for Ineffective Coping* related to prolonged hospitalization

8. Which of the following explanations by the nurse to reinforce the patient's preoperative education for a loop ostomy would be correct?
   1. "You will have a stoma in the middle of your abdomen that will constantly drain liquid stool."
   2. "You will have a looped bag system to collect stool from your stoma."
   3. "You will have a loop of bowel on your abdomen, but it will not drain stool."
   4. "You will have a loop of bowel on your abdomen that can be returned to your abdomen after your bowel has healed."

9. Which of the following dietary instructions is most important to include in the plan of care to prevent complications for a patient with an ileostomy?
   1. "Drink lots of fluids to prevent dehydration."
   2. "Avoid fruits and vegetables to prevent diarrhea."
   3. "Avoid milk products to prevent gas."
   4. "Eat plenty of fiber to prevent constipation."

10. A patient is concerned about ileostomy odor. Which of the following responses by the nurse would be best?
    1. "A teaspoon of baking soda in your pouch will absorb all the odor."
    2. "The plastic your pouch is made of is odor-proof. You shouldn't have to worry about odor as long as you don't have a leak."
    3. "Effluent from an ileostomy has no odor. It is colostomies that can smell bad from time to time."
    4. "Changing your pouch and face plate daily will help prevent odor."

11. The nurse is counseling a patient with frequent anal fissures and a history of constipation. Which of the following indicates that teaching has been effective?
    1. "I guess there isn't much I can do except seek pain relief whenever I have a fissure."
    2. "It is important that I not ignore the urge to have a bowel movement."
    3. "Decreasing the amount of fluid I drink each day will reduce stool frequency and subsequent irritation."
    4. "Narcotic pain medications are probably needed to help with this condition."

35 Nursing Care of Patients With Liver, Pancreatic, and Gallbladder Disorders

VOCABULARY

Match the following terms with the appropriate description.

1. _____ Ascites
2. _____ Asterixis
3. _____ Cirrhosis
4. _____ Encephalopathy
5. _____ Fetor hepaticus
6. _____ Hepatorenal syndrome
7. _____ Hepatitis
8. _____ Jaundice
9. _____ Portal hypertension
10. _____ Pancreatectomy
11. _____ Steatorrhea
12. _____ Varices

1. Yellowing of the sclerae and skin from excess bilirubin
2. Removal of all or part of the pancreas
3. Liver flap
4. Fluid in the abdomen from decreased albumin
5. Neurologic changes from excess ammonia
6. Weakened, swollen veins
7. Foul breath
8. Fatty, foul-smelling stools
9. Increased pressure in the portal circulation
10. Scarring and hardening of the liver from inflammation
11. Oliguria and sodium retention without kidney defects
12. Inflammation of the liver cells

LIVER

Fill in the crossword with terms related to the liver.

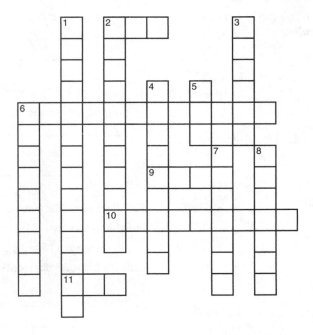

Across

2. Abbreviation for serum hepatitis
6. Visible veins around umbilicus
9. Abbreviation for liver shunt
10. Liver flap
11. Abbreviation for infectious hepatitis

Down

1. Confusion and coma are symptoms
2. This syndrome causes oliguria
3. Abdomen circulation
4. Liver inflammation
5. Abbreviation for liver location
6. Progressive, irreversible replacement of liver tissue with scar tissue
7. Collection of fluid in peritoneal cavity
8. Dilated esophageal veins

GALLBLADDER

Match the following terms with the appropriate description.

1. _____Cholecystitis
2. _____Cholesterol
3. _____Flatulence
4. _____Murphy's sign
5. _____Bilirubin
6. _____Extracorporeal shock wave lithotripsy (ESWL)
7. _____T-tube
8. _____Laparoscopic cholecystectomy
9. _____Chenodeoxycholic acid
10. _____Choledochoscopy

1. Pigment from the breakdown of hemoglobin in red blood cells
2. Dissolves cholesterol gallstones
3. Use of an endoscope to explore the common bile duct
4. Inflammation of the gallbladder
5. Inability to take a deep breath when fingers are pressed under liver margin
6. Substance found in gallstones
7. Intestinal gas expelled via the rectum
8. A procedure that shatters gallstones using sound waves
9. A surgical drain used to ensure that bile drains freely from the gallbladder after surgery
10. Removal of the gallbladder through a small abdominal incision

PANCREAS

In the space on the left, write N or A to indicate whether the assessment finding is normal or abnormal. If the finding is abnormal, indicate the possible (liver-, gallbladder-, or pancreas-related) cause for the finding.

1. _____Serum glucose >150 mg%

2. _____Serum amylase >500 international unit/L

3. _____Serum lipase = 15 unit/L

4. _____Pleural effusion

5. _____Blood pressure and pulse 15% from patient's baseline

6. _____Serum albumin <3.2 g/dL

7. _____Positive Cullen's sign

8. _____Urinary output <30 mL/hr

9. _____Positive Chvostek's sign

10. _____Foul-smelling, fatty stools

CRITICAL THINKING

Read the following case study and answer the questions.

Ms. Bettina Smythe has been diagnosed with hepatic encephalopathy secondary to cirrhosis. During the admission process, the nurse notes the following findings: abdomen grossly distended, yellow sclerae and skin, multiple bruises, and pitting edema of the lower extremities. The nurse also notes that Ms. Smythe is irritable and has difficulty answering questions and appears to doze off frequently during the interview. The nurse observes that Ms. Smythe scratches her arms and legs frequently. Her laboratory data indicate that her serum bilirubin, ammonia, and prothrombin time are elevated and that her serum albumin, total protein, and potassium are below normal.

1. What data support the diagnosis of cirrhosis?

_____

_____

_____

_____

2. What data suggest that Ms. Smythe has hepatic encephalopathy? What other evidence might be observed?

_____

_____

_____

_____

_____

3. Why is Ms. Smythe exhibiting pitting edema and abdominal distention? _____

_____

_____

_____

_____

4. What medical treatments can the nurse expect will be ordered for hepatic encephalopathy? _____

_____

_____

_____

Two days after Ms. Smythe was admitted, there is bright red blood in her emesis. Ms. Smythe also reports feeling cold, and her pulse is 115 beats per minute and thready. The nurse calls for help and places Ms. Smythe on her side.

5. What further treatment can be anticipated for Ms. Smythe?

_____

_____

_____

_____

6. What observations should be made to detect bleeding from lack of clotting factors? _____

_____

_____

7. What nursing measures can be provided to help Ms. Smythe maintain her fluid balance? _____

_____

_____

8. What should Ms. Smythe be taught about taking acetaminophen (Tylenol)? Why? _____

_____

_____

_____

WORD SEARCH

Gallbladder

```
C  W  J  V  L  S  U  P  O  M  C  Q  R  S  M  R  W  S  M  X
W  D  Q  I  Y  W  A  W  E  W  V  H  U  L  U  I  K  W  V  S
O  E  Y  L  V  X  Z  B  S  N  L  S  W  V  F  N  V  P  Q  R
W  V  S  D  N  O  U  C  T  E  A  S  X  U  W  I  F  L  U  S
F  T  K  T  J  G  Z  H  H  Q  E  C  W  P  S  B  I  N  G  V
L  -  Q  Y  B  C  D  O  H  V  U  X  R  C  H  U  P  Z  L  X
A  T  K  M  K  H  D  L  G  K  W  H  Z  K  U  R  A  Z  B  F
T  U  F  U  C  C  F  E  Q  X  P  X  C  G  O  I  C  E  M  S
U  B  Y  R  Y  P  O  C  S  O  H  C  O  D  E  L  O  H  C  Q
L  E  H  P  B  E  Y  Y  L  Z  M  D  M  X  O  I  P  L  L  K
E  G  E  H  D  K  V  S  P  O  G  M  P  Q  D  B  O  C  S  D
N  N  P  Y  V  N  X  T  B  Q  M  B  A  J  B  R  I  S  D  L
C  P  S  '  Y  J  T  I  G  N  A  A  P  C  E  O  V  K  N  R
E  I  F  S  M  T  O  T  F  L  O  E  W  T  V  I  W  H  V  J
U  S  L  S  O  L  B  I  Z  P  P  X  S  C  O  D  H  N  J  X
S  X  O  I  O  M  E  S  G  L  S  E  W  P  Y  M  X  U  W  O
R  D  J  G  S  V  Z  M  B  B  L  R  H  J  Z  B  C  E  A  T
M  R  C  N  G  Y  A  T  H  O  R  Z  Z  F  V  U  I  P  Z  Z
J  O  R  L  P  Q  F  Q  H  N  H  Y  B  N  O  Y  S  T  C  W
L  Q  N  L  S  U  W  C  F  S  R  V  L  O  I  D  O  S  R  U
```

Write the definition of the word and then find the word on the preceding figure.

1. Bilirubin _____
2. Choledochoscopy _____
3. Cholesterol _____
4. Cholecystitis _____
5. ESWL _____

6. Flatulence _____
7. Murphy's sign _____
8. T-tube _____
9. Ursodiol _____

REVIEW QUESTIONS—CONTENT REVIEW

Choose the best answer unless directed otherwise.

1. Which of the following precautions will protect the nurse who is caring for the patient with hepatitis B?
   1. Reverse isolation
   2. Standard precautions
   3. Respiratory precautions
   4. Enteric precautions

2. Acute liver failure is most often caused by which of the following?
   1. Antibiotic use
   2. Daily vitamins
   3. Alcohol use
   4. Acetaminophen (Tylenol) overdose

3. Which of the following is a treatment for bleeding esophageal varices? **Select all that apply.**
   1. Variceal ligation (banding)
   2. Octreotide (Sandostatin) intravenous (IV)
   3. Soft diet
   4. Sclerotherapy

4. Which of the following is a nonsurgical intervention for the management of biliary colic?
   1. Encouraging a high-fat diet
   2. Administering vitamin K
   3. Administering chenodeoxycholic acid (Chenodiol)
   4. Administering propantheline (Pro-Banthine)

5. Patients with a history of pancreatic disease commonly have a history of which of the following?
   1. High-protein diet
   2. Very-low-fat diet
   3. Excessive alcohol consumption
   4. Excessive intake of vitamin C

6. Patients with acute pancreatitis frequently describe their pain as which of the following?
   1. Dull, boring, beginning in the mid epigastrium and radiating to the back
   2. Knifelike, centered in the left lower quadrant
   3. Burning, focused over the left flank and radiating to the shoulder
   4. Sharp, severe pain that begins in the right upper quadrant

REVIEW QUESTIONS—TEST PREPARATION

Choose the best answer unless directed otherwise.

7. A patient with ascites is placed on a low-sodium diet. The nurse knows that diet teaching has been successful if the patient selects which of the following meals?
   1. Cottage cheese and peaches with tomato juice
   2. Frankfurter on a bun with pickle relish and skim milk
   3. Baked chicken, white rice, and apple juice
   4. Turkey and lettuce sandwich on whole-wheat bread with tomato soup

8. Which of the following are risk factors for gallbladder disease? **Select all that apply.**
   1. Male gender
   2. Obesity
   3. Multiple pregnancies
   4. Age 40 or older
   5. Fasting
   6. Diabetes mellitus

9. Which of the following instructions should be given to the patient with portal hypertension? **Select all that apply.**
   1. Cough and deep breathe every 2 hours.
   2. Avoid straining to have a bowel movement.
   3. Avoid heavy lifting
   4. Increase fluid intake.
   5. Take vitamin K supplements.

10. A patient with cirrhosis has asterixis and fetor hepaticus and is confused. The nurse recognizes these as symptoms of which complication?
    1. Hepatic encephalopathy
    2. Hepatorenal syndrome
    3. Portal hypertension
    4. Ascites

unit NINE

Understanding the Urinary System

CHECKLIST FOR LEARNING SUCCESS

Review of Anatomy and Physiology and Aging Changes	Major Disorders	Nursing Assessment	Diagnostic Tests	Interventions	Common Medications
❑ Kidneys	❑ Incontinence	❑ Medical history	❑ Urinalysis	❑ Urinary catheters	❑ Diuretics
❑ Urine	❑ Urinary retention	❑ Medications	❑ Urine culture	❑ Lithotripsy	❑ Sodium polystyrene sulfonate (Kayexalate)
❑ Elimination of urine	❑ Urinary tract infections	❑ Vital signs	❑ Blood urea nitrogen	❑ Hemodialysis	❑ Phosphate binder
❑ Aging effects	❑ Urological obstructions	❑ Physical examination	❑ Creatinine	❑ Peritoneal dialysis	
	❑ Tumors	❑ Intake and output	❑ Creatinine clearance	❑ Continuous renal replacement therapy	
	❑ Polycystic kidney disease	❑ Daily weights	❑ Kidneys-ureter-bladder	❑ Urinary diversion	
	❑ Chronic renal diseases		❑ Intravenous (IV) pyelogram		
	❑ Acute kidney injury		❑ Cystoscopy and pyelogram		
	❑ Chronic kidney disease				
	❑ Kidney transplantation				

36

Urinary System Function, Assessment, and Therapeutic Measures

VOCABULARY

Match the term for an abnormality of the urine or urination with the correct description.

1. _____ Hematuria
2. _____ Dysuria
3. _____ Nocturia
4. _____ Oliguria
5. _____ Enuresis
6. _____ Anuria
7. _____ Polyuria
8. _____ Pyuria

1. Painful urination
2. Decreased urine output (<400 mL per 24 hours)
3. Blood in the urine
4. Voiding during the night
5. Excessive urination (>2000 mL per 24 hours)
6. Absence of urination
7. Presence of pus in the urine
8. Bedwetting

ANATOMY REVIEW

Label the parts of the kidney and nephron.

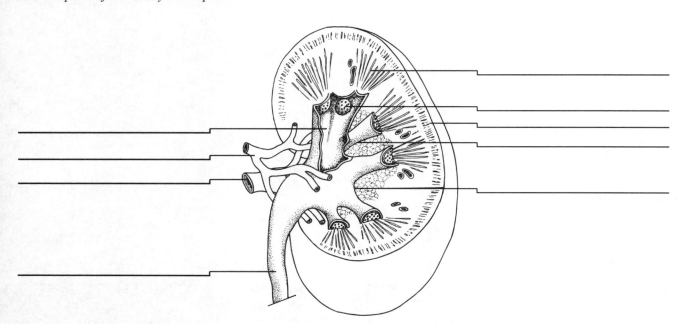

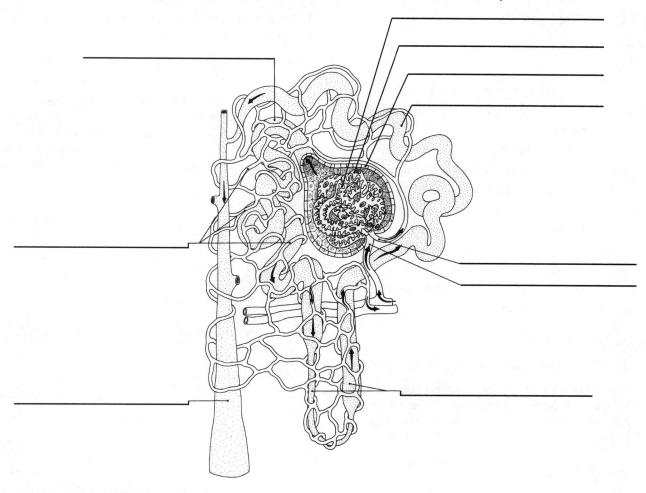

SAMPLE URINALYSIS RESULTS

Review the urinalysis results of the following three patients and determine the most likely cause of the abnormal results.

	Patient A	Patient B	Patient C
Color	Yellow	Dark amber	Yellow-green
Character	Cloudy	Concentrated	Clear
Glucose	Negative	Negative	Negative
Bilirubin	Negative	Negative	2+
Ketones	Small	Negative	Negative
Specific gravity (1.010–1.025)	1.024	1.035	1.025
Hemoglobin	Small	Negative	Negative
pH (5.0–9.0)	6.0	5.2	5.5
Protein	100	Negative	Negative
Urobilinogen (0.2–1.0)	0.2	0.2	0.2
Nitrite	Positive	Negative	Negative
Urine microscopic casts	White blood cell (WBC), red blood cell (RBC)	Negative	Negative
WBCs (0–4 HPF)	400	4	1
RBCs (0–4 HPF)	90	2	2
Crystals	Negative	2	Negative
Amorphous	Negative	Negative	Negative
Epithelial cells (negative)	3	Negative	2
Bacteria (negative)	4+	Negative	Negative
Yeast (negative)	Negative	Negative	Negative

Patient A: _____

Patient B: _____

Patient C: _____

RENAL DIAGNOSTIC TESTS

Label each statement as true or false and correct the false statements.

1. _____ An x-ray of the renal structures after injection of a radiopaque dye into the venous system is called a renal ultrasound.

2. _____ A diagnostic test in which sound waves are used to outline the structure of the kidney is a pyelogram.

3. _____ A urine sample that is cultured to determine the kind of bacteria it contains is called a creatinine clearance urine test.

4. _____ A diagnostic test in which the inside of the bladder is visualized is called a cystoscopy.

5. _____ The radiopaque dye used when doing diagnostic tests of the renal system is harmless.

CRITICAL THINKING

Read the following case studies and answer the questions.

Mrs. Bohke is a 64-year-old female patient admitted to the hospital with a diagnosis of pneumonia. During her stay, she tells the nurse she has trouble getting to the bathroom on time and often dribbles before she can get to the bathroom.

1. What type of urinary incontinence does she have?

_____

_____

_____

2. What teaching could be done to help her decrease her incontinence? _____

_____

_____

Mrs. Simmon is a 79-year-old woman with a fractured hip and a previous cerebrovascular accident (CVA). She has poor vision but is alert mentally. The nurse finds her lying in bed in a puddle of urine, crying. She explains that she was unable to find her call light. The nurse finds it lying on the floor out of her reach.

3. What kind of incontinence did Mrs. Simmon experience?

_____

_____

_____

_____

4. What actions should the nurse take to ensure that this does not happen again? _____

_____

_____

_____

5. When caring for a patient with incontinence, is it helpful to decrease fluid intake? Why or why not? _____

_____

_____

_____

_____

REVIEW QUESTIONS—CONTENT REVIEW

Choose the best answer unless otherwise directed.

1. Which of the following is secreted when the blood level of oxygen decreases?
   1. Erythropoietin
   2. Renin
   3. Angiotensin II
   4. Vitamin D

2. Urea is a nitrogenous waste product from the metabolism of which of the following?
   1. Nucleic acids
   2. Amino acids
   3. Muscle tissue
   4. Carbohydrates

3. The kidneys are located behind which of the following structures?
   1. Spinal column
   2. Diaphragm
   3. Peritoneum
   4. Inferior vena cava

4. The renal pyramids make up which kidney structure?
   1. Renal cortex
   2. Renal medulla
   3. Renal pelvis
   4. Renal fascia

5. The process of tubular resorption takes place in which of the following parts of the kidney?
   1. From the glomerulus to Bowman's capsule
   2. From the afferent arteriole to the efferent arteriole
   3. From the peritubular capillaries to the glomerulus
   4. From the renal tubule to the peritubular capillaries

6. Where is urine formed?
   1. Nephrons
   2. Ureters
   3. Urethra
   4. Bladder

7. Which of the following are functions of the kidney?
   Select all that apply.
   1. Maintaining acid–base balance
   2. Removal of waste products
   3. Regulation of the blood volume
   4. Regulation of electrolytes
   5. Removal of CO_2
   6. Production of erythropoietin

REVIEW QUESTIONS—TEST PREPARATION

Choose the best answer unless otherwise directed.

8. When collecting a urine specimen on a newly admitted female patient, the nurse should take which of the following actions?
   1. Direct the patient to wash perineum before collecting the urine specimen.
   2. Have the patient void, throw that urine away, and then collect another specimen.
   3. Obtain the last voided urine of the day.
   4. Direct the patient to drink at least three glasses of water.

9. A patient's urinalysis results show the following findings: urine, dark amber; bacteria, small amount; nitrite, negative; specific gravity, 1.035. Which of the following is the best explanation for these results?
   1. Dehydration
   2. Urinary tract infection
   3. Contamination of the specimen from bacteria on the perineum
   4. Contamination from menstruation

10. Which of the following diagnostic test results would the nurse evaluate as being related to renal disease?
    Select all that apply.
    1. Hematocrit: 39%
    2. Potassium: 4.0 mEq/L
    3. Uric acid: 2 ng/dL
    4. Creatinine: 3 mg/dL
    5. BUN: 35 mg/dL
    6. Urine specific gravity: 1.020

11. A patient is scheduled for a pyelogram with contrast. When giving care, the nurse should recognize that restriction of which of the following is part of the preparation for a pyelogram?
    1. Salt intake
    2. Fluid intake
    3. Use of tobacco
    4. Physical activities

12. The patient is scheduled for a cystoscopy. Which of the following is the most important nursing care after this kind of surgery?
    1. Measuring urine output
    2. Monitoring daily weights
    3. Observing for symptoms of acute kidney injury
    4. Limiting fluid intake

13. A patient, age 48, has urge incontinence. When assessing the patient, the nurse would expect to find which of the following symptoms?
    1. Patient is unable to reach the bathroom in time and ends up urinating in underwear.
    2. Patient is incontinent of small amounts of urine when coughs, sneezes, or bears down.
    3. Patient is incontinent of urine when has many responsibilities and becomes overloaded.
    4. Patient is incontinent because unable to tell when needs to urinate and unable to control urination.

14. Which of the following actions should the nurse take to prevent development of a urinary tract infection in a patient who has a urinary catheter inserted?
    1. Limit fluid intake to 2000 mL per 24 hours to decrease the flow of urine, which can result in increased contamination.
    2. Wash the perineum with an antibacterial soap three times per 24 hours.
    3. Keep catheter securely taped to the patient, preventing back-and-forth motion of the catheter.
    4. Empty the urinary catheter bag only when needed to prevent contamination of the exit spout.

15. Which of the following actions should the nurse take for a patient who has total urinary incontinence?
    1. Give patient cranberry juice to keep the urine acidic.
    2. Ensure that patient has ready access to the urinal.
    3. Teach patient how to do Kegel exercises to increase perineal tone.
    4. Apply an adult incontinence brief to catch urine and change when necessary.

37

Nursing Care of Patients With Disorders of the Urinary System

VOCABULARY

Fill in the blank with the correct term.

1. _____ is inflammation of the urethra.
2. _____ is inflammation of the bladder.
3. _____ is inflammation of the kidney.
4. Surgical repair of the urethra is called _____.
5. Kidney stones are also called _____.
6. _____ is surgical incision into the kidney to remove a stone.
7. Unrelieved obstruction of the urinary tract can lead to _____.
8. A _____ tube may be inserted directly into the kidney pelvis to drain urine.
9. Surgical removal of a kidney is called a _____.
10. Thickening and hardening of the renal blood vessels is called _____.

URINARY TRACT INFECTIONS.

Answer the following questions.

1. What is the usual cause of urinary tract infections (UTIs) in women? _____
   _____

2. What is the usual cause of UTIs in men? _____
   _____

3. What advice regarding fluids should be given to patients who are susceptible to UTIs? _____
   _____

4. What is the single most important thing a patient with a history of UTIs should be taught? _____
   _____

5. Compare cystitis (bladder infection) versus pyelonephritis (kidney infection) by filling out the following table.

Things to Compare	Cystitis	Pyelonephritis
Symptoms	_____	_____
	_____	_____
	_____	_____
	_____	_____
	_____	_____
Urinalysis Results	_____	_____
	_____	_____
	_____	_____
	_____	_____
	_____	_____
Prognosis	_____	_____

URINARY TRACT OBSTRUCTIONS

Answer the following questions.

1. What is the most common symptom of cancer of the bladder? _____
   _____

2. What is the most common risk factor for cancer of the bladder? _____

3. What is the most common symptom of cancer of the kidney? _____

4. What does the urine look like when a patient has an ileal conduit? _____

5. What nursing care should be provided for a patient with an ileal conduit? _____

6. What is the most important care that should be given a patient with a kidney stone? _____

7. What teaching should be done for the patient to prevent further stone formation if the stone is composed of calcium oxalate? Uric acid? _____

CRITICAL THINKING

Read the following case study and answer the questions.

Mrs. Zins is a 27-year-old woman who has had Type 1 diabetes mellitus for more than 20 years. Recently she has begun having incidents of hypoglycemia, she is edematous, and her blood pressure has elevated. She is admitted to the hospital for diagnosis and treatment of probable chronic kidney disease.

History: Subjective Data

States that she has been exhausted lately and her skin is itchy.
States that she has been very irritable and her husband says she is difficult to live with.

Physical: Objective Data

BP 194/104 mm Hg, P 98 beats per minute, R 22 per minute, T 98.4°F (36.9°C)
Jugular vein distention present at 45 degrees
Generalized edema throughout body, including periorbital edema
Pitting edema of feet and ankles
Weight gain of 20 pounds in 2 months
Skin very dry, flaky

Diagnostic Tests

Fasting blood sugar: 56 mg/100 L
Serum sodium: 145 mEq/L
Serum creatinine: 5.4 mg/100 L
Serum potassium: 5.9 mEq/L
Uric acid: 8.2 ng/dL

Hemoglobin (Hgb): 7.2 g/100 mL
Hematocrit (Hct): 22%

1. Mrs. Zins has been having incidents of hypoglycemia. Why is this happening? _____

2. With Mrs. Zins present blood sugar of 56, what kind of juice should the nurse give her? _____

3. How does diabetes cause chronic kidney disease? _____

4. Is there anything Mrs. Zins could have done to decrease the possibility of developing chronic kidney disease? _____

5. Identify two nursing diagnoses that would be appropriate for Mrs. Zins based on her assessment. _____

6. What diagnostic test was most indicative of chronic kidney disease for Mrs. Zins? _____

7. Why is Mrs. Zins anemic? _____

8. What would be the three most important areas for nursing data collection for Mrs. Zins related to her chronic kidney disease? _____

9. What kind of diet will Mrs. Zins most likely receive? _____

CHRONIC KIDNEY DISEASE

Fill in the signs and symptoms of kidney disease under the body systems on the figure that follows.

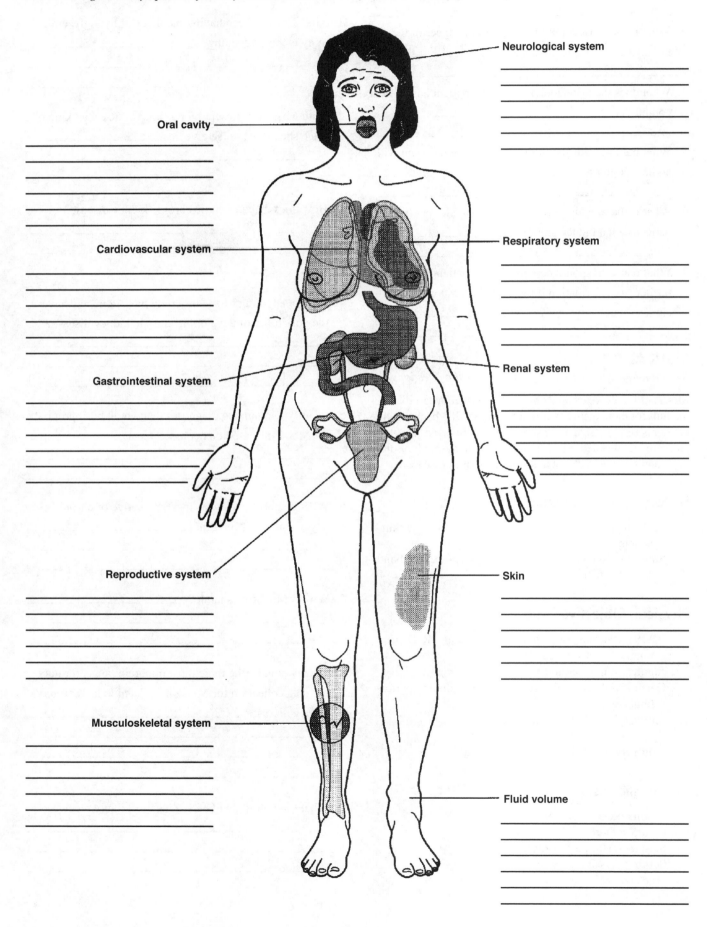

Neurological system

Oral cavity

Respiratory system

Cardiovascular system

Renal system

Gastrointestinal system

Reproductive system

Skin

Musculoskeletal system

Fluid volume

REVIEW QUESTIONS—CONTENT REVIEW

Choose the best answer unless directed otherwise.

1. Which of the following is the most common symptom of cancer of the bladder?
   1. Nocturia
   2. Dysuria
   3. Urinary retention
   4. Hematuria

2. When examining the patient, the nurse notes the following diagnostic tests on the patient's chart. Which of the following diagnostic tests results is most indicative of acute kidney injury?
   1. BUN: 80 mg/100 mL (8–25 mg/100 L)
   2. 24-hour creatinine clearance: 5 mL/min (100 mL/min)
   3. Uric acid: 8 ng/dL (2.5–5.5 ng/dL)
   4. Serum creatinine: 1.7 mg/100 L (0.5–1.5 mg/100 L)

3. Which of the following foods should the patient be taught to avoid for a kidney stone composed of calcium oxalate?
   1. Bread
   2. Beer
   3. Beef
   4. Beans

REVIEW QUESTIONS—TEST PREPARATION

Choose the best answer unless directed otherwise.

4. Postoperatively, the nurse notes the presence of mucus in the urinary drainage. Which of the following actions should the nurse take?
   1. Notify the health care provider (HCP).
   2. Collect a urine specimen for culture and sensitivity.
   3. Measure the specific gravity of the urine.
   4. Recognize that this is a normal occurrence.

5. Which of the following is the most significant sign of acute kidney injury that the nurse should recognize during data collection?
   1. A rise in blood pressure
   2. An elevation in body temperature
   3. A decrease in urine output
   4. An increase in urine specific gravity

6. A patient with acute kidney injury has been instructed to limit potassium intake. The nurse recognizes that teaching has been effective if the patient chooses which of the following snacks? **Select all that apply.**
   1. Chocolates
   2. An orange
   3. Grapefruit juice
   4. A gelatin dessert
   5. Cranberry juice

7. A patient with severe right flank pain, general weakness, and fever is hospitalized. The patient has a history of recurrent urinary tract infection, and renal calculi are suspected. On the second hospital day, the patient's urine output drops to 300 mL/24 hr, and the patient has distention and pain in the suprapubic area. The nurse would suspect which of the following to be the most likely cause for this sudden change?
   1. Sudden decreased renal perfusion
   2. Inadequate fluid intake
   3. Interstitial fluid shift
   4. Urinary tract obstruction

8. Which of the following is appropriate patient teaching to obtain a midstream urine specimen for culture and sensitivity?
   1. A second-voided specimen is preferred.
   2. The specimen should be collected early in the morning.
   3. The patient should begin voiding, collect the specimen, and then finish voiding in the toilet.
   4. A 24-hour urine specimen is needed; the first void should be discarded.

9. A patient is admitted with chronic kidney disease. The patient has a potassium level of 6.4 mEq/L, is placed on a cardiac monitor and given sodium polystyrene sulfonate (kayexalate) by retention enema. Which of the following is the most significant symptom that the nurse should recognize during data collection?
   1. Diarrhea
   2. Irregular heart rhythm
   3. Increased blood pressure
   4. Increased respiratory rate

10. The nursing diagnosis of *Excess Fluid Volume* is made for a patient with chronic kidney disease. Which of the following information is most important for the nurse to collect for this patient based on the nursing diagnosis?
    1. Intake and output
    2. Vital signs
    3. Daily weight
    4. Skin turgor

11. A patient with newly diagnosed chronic kidney disease has elevated sodium, potassium, and serum creatinine levels. When the breakfast tray is served, there is a glass of orange juice on it. Which of the following actions should the nurse take?
    1. Encourage the patient to drink the orange juice for vitamin C to help fight the infection.
    2. Remove the orange juice from the tray because it is high in potassium.
    3. Give the patient a smaller glass of orange juice because the patient is on a fluid restriction.
    4. Check the kind of diet the patient is on to determine any restrictions.

12. A patient goes to surgery for fistula creation for dialysis. The patient asks why it needs to be done. Which of the following is the best explanation by the nurse on the advantages of a fistula over a two-tailed subclavian catheter?
    1. "There is a larger blood flow, and dialysis is more efficient."
    2. "There is less risk of clotting with the fistula."
    3. "It is easier to access the fistula than the two-tailed subclavian."
    4. "It is less likely to be damaged by trauma."

13. After hemodialysis, which of the following nursing interventions is imperative for the nurse to carry out? **Select all that apply.**
    1. Document stool output.
    2. Weigh the patient.
    3. Check for jugular vein distention.
    4. Obtain vital signs.
    5. Allow patient to rest.

14. The patient has a permanent peritoneal catheter inserted and is begun on continuous ambulatory peritoneal dialysis (CAPD). The patient asks how it works. Which of the following would be the best explanation of how this type of dialysis works?
    1. The peritoneum allows solutes in the dialysate to pass into the intravascular system.
    2. The peritoneum acts as a semipermeable membrane through which solutes move by diffusion and osmosis.
    3. The presence of excess metabolites causes increased permeability of the peritoneum and allows excess fluid to drain.
    4. The peritoneum permits diffusion of metabolites from the intravascular to the interstitial space.

15. A patient on dialysis has a severe cerebrovascular accident and is now semicomatose. His family decides that dialysis should be stopped. He is sent home with his daughter and hospice to die. As part of discharge planning, his daughter should be taught to expect which of the following symptoms of untreated end-stage renal failure?
    1. Polyuria, pruritus, and extreme irritability
    2. Dehydration with sunken eyeballs and oliguria
    3. Edema, possible convulsions, then coma
    4. Decreased respiratory rate and cyanosis

16. A patient is admitted who was involved in a motor vehicle accident resulting in trauma to the abdomen and back. The patient has a ruptured spleen and probable trauma to the kidneys. For which of the following changes in the patient's urine should the nurse observe?
    1. Dysuria
    2. Pyuria
    3. Polyuria
    4. Hematuria

17. A patient is admitted with symptoms of a recent weight gain, pitting edema of his feet, jugular vein distension, and lung crackles. Which of the following nursing diagnoses is most appropriate for this patient's plan of care?
    1. Deficient Fluid Volume
    2. Excess Fluid Volume
    3. Imbalanced Nutrition: More Than Body Requirements
    4. Noncompliance

unit TEN

Understanding the Endocrine System

CHECKLIST FOR LEARNING SUCCESS

Review of Anatomy and Physiology and Aging Changes	Major Disorders	Nursing Assessment	Diagnostic Tests	Interventions	Common Medications
❑ Antidiuretic hormone	❑ Diabetes insipidus	❑ History	❑ 24-hour urine	❑ Interventions for fluid imbalances	❑ Hormone replacement
❑ Growth hormone	❑ Syndrome of inappropriate antidiuretic hormone secretion (SIADH)	❑ Fluid balance	❑ Hormone levels	❑ Pre- and post-thyroidectomy care	❑ Calcium
❑ Thyroid-stimulating hormone		❑ Mood, affect	❑ Stimulation tests		❑ Calcitonin
❑ Adrenocorticotropic hormone		❑ Exophthalmos	❑ Suppression tests	❑ Pre- and post-hypophysectomy care	❑ Thyroid hormone
❑ T_3 and T_4	❑ Acromegaly	❑ Skin	❑ Thyroid scan	❑ Teaching related to self-care	❑ Insulin
❑ Calcitonin	❑ Hypothyroidism	❑ Vital signs	❑ Blood glucose	❑ Diabetes education	❑ Oral hypoglycemic agents
❑ Parathyroid hormone	❑ Hyperthyroidism	❑ Tremor	❑ Glycohemoglobin		
❑ Glucagon	❑ Goiter	❑ Polyuria, polydipsia, polyphagia	❑ Glucose tolerance test		
❑ Insulin	❑ Thyroid cancer	❑ Self-monitoring of blood glucose (SMBG)	❑ Ultrasound		
❑ Norepinephrine	❑ Hypoparathyroidism		❑ Biopsy		
❑ Epinephrine	❑ Hyperparathyroidism	❑ Knowledge of self-care			
❑ Aldosterone	❑ Pheochromocytoma				
❑ Cortisol	❑ Addison's disease				
❑ Aging changes	❑ Cushing's syndrome				
	❑ Diabetes mellitus				
	❑ Reactive hypoglycemia				

38

Endocrine System Function and Assessment

VOCABULARY

Complete the following sentences with the appropriate words.

1. Glucose is converted to _____ for storage.

2. High blood glucose is called _____.

3. Emotional tone is called _____.

4. Bulging eyes, or _____, is a symptom of hyperthyroidism.

5. Hormone secretion is regulated through a _____ system.

HORMONES

Match each hormone with its function. Use each number only once.

1. _____ Antidiuretic hormone (ADH)

2. _____ Oxytocin

3. _____ Thyroid-stimulating hormone

4. _____ Adrenocorticotropic hormone

5. _____ Growth hormone (GH)

6. _____ Prolactin

7. _____ Follicle-stimulating hormone

8. _____ Luteinizing hormone

9. _____ Thyroxine

10. _____ Calcitonin

11. _____ Parathyroid hormone (PTH)

12. _____ Epinephrine

13. _____ Norepinephrine

14. _____ Cortisol

15. _____ Aldosterone

16. _____ Insulin

17. _____ Glucagon

1. Stimulates growth and secretions of the thyroid gland
2. Increases glucose uptake by cells and glycogen storage in the liver
3. Decreases the resorption of calcium from bones; lowers blood calcium level
4. Increases the use of fats and amino acids for energy and has an anti-inflammatory effect
5. Stimulates mitosis and protein synthesis
6. Increases heart rate and force of contraction
7. Causes vasoconstriction throughout the body
8. Increases secretion of cortisol by the adrenal cortex
9. Increases energy production for a normal metabolic rate
10. Directly increases water reabsorption by the kidneys
11. In men, stimulates secretion of testosterone
12. Increases the conversion of glycogen to glucose in the liver between meals
13. Initiates milk production in the mammary glands
14. Increases the resorption of calcium from bones; raises blood calcium level
15. Increases the resorption of sodium by the kidneys
16. In women, initiates development of ova in ovaries
17. Causes contraction of the myometrium during labor

ENDOCRINE GLANDS AND HORMONES

Label the figure with the glands of the endocrine system. List the hormone(s) secreted by each gland.

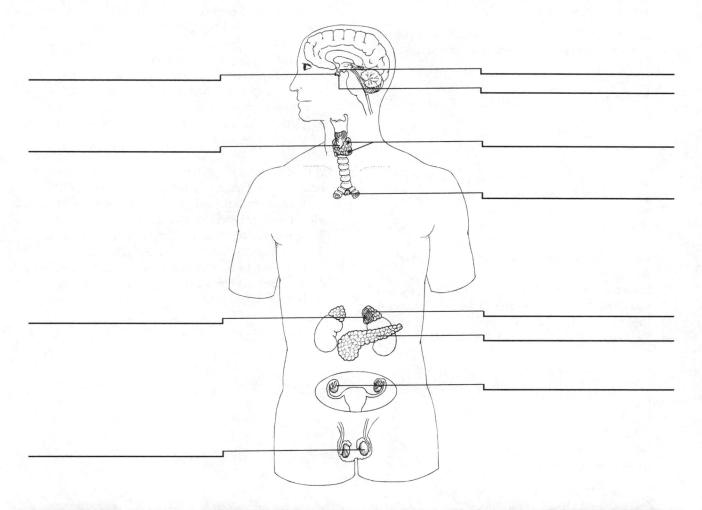

REVIEW QUESTIONS—CONTENT REVIEW

Choose the best answer unless directed otherwise.

1. Which two hormones help regulate the blood calcium level?
   1. Insulin and glucagon
   2. Calcitonin and PTH
   3. Thyroxine and epinephrine
   4. Cortisol and aldosterone

2. Which hormone is most important for day-to-day regulation of metabolic rate?
   1. Insulin
   2. Epinephrine
   3. GH
   4. Thyroxine

3. What happens when aldosterone increases the reabsorption of sodium ions by the kidneys?
   1. Water is also reabsorbed back to the blood.
   2. Bicarbonate ions are excreted in urine.
   3. More water is excreted in urine.
   4. Potassium ions are also reabsorbed back into the blood.

4. Which of the following hormones has an anti-inflammatory effect?
   1. Epinephrine
   2. Cortisol
   3. Aldosterone
   4. Thyroxine

REVIEW QUESTIONS—TEST PREPARATION

Choose the best answer unless directed otherwise.

5. Which of the following hormones help maintain blood volume and blood pressure? **Select all that apply.**
   1. Thyroxine
   2. Glucagon
   3. Aldosterone
   4. Cortisol
   5. ADH
   6. Insulin

6. A patient is completing a 24-hour urine test. What should the nurse do to complete the test at the end of the 24 hours?
   1. Have the patient void exactly 24 hours after the test was begun and discard the specimen.
   2. Save the last specimen and send it in a separate container.
   3. Have the patient void exactly 24 hours after the test was begun, and add this urine to the remainder of the specimen.
   4. Send only the specimen voided at 24 hours.

7. A female patient is admitted to the hospital with hyperthyroidism. What related assessment should the nurse perform?
   1. Check the patient's heart rate.
   2. Palpate the thyroid gland for enlargement.
   3. Do a capillary blood glucose level.
   4. Observe for a "buffalo hump" on the patient's back.

8. A patient asks the nurse, "My doctor told me my thyroid scan showed a 'cold spot.' What does that mean?" Which of the following responses by the nurse is best?
   1. "That means you have cancer of the thyroid gland."
   2. "Cold spots are areas that have no living tissue."
   3. "A cold spot is an area that did not pick up the radioactive material they injected."
   4. "It doesn't mean anything. A cold spot is just part of your thyroid gland."

9. A patient with a suspected autoimmune disease has laboratory work ordered, including a cortisol level. The nurse recognizes that cortisol is responsible for which of the following? **Select all that apply.**
   1. Stimulates conversion of triglycerides to glucose.
   2. Stimulates the storage of excess glucose.
   3. Increases the breakdown of lipids to fatty acids.
   4. Increases the breakdown of proteins to amino acids.
   5. Blocks the effect of histamine.

Nursing Care of Patients With Endocrine Disorders

39

VOCABULARY

Use the following terms to fill in the blanks.

Amenorrhea	Myxedema
Dysphagia	Nocturia
Ectopic	Polydipsia
Euthyroid	Polyuria
Goiter	Pheochromocytoma

1. A normally functioning thyroid gland produces a _____ state.
2. Enlargement of the thyroid gland is called a _____.
3. Excessive thirst is called _____.
4. Excessive urination is called _____.
5. A _____ is a tumor of the adrenal medulla.
6. Difficulty swallowing is called _____.
7. Untreated hypothyroidism can lead to _____ coma.
8. _____ is the word for getting up to void during the night.
9. Absence of menses is called _____.
10. Sometimes hormones are produced outside the endocrine gland in a/an _____ site.

HORMONES

Match the disorder in column 1 to a hormone imbalance in column 2 and signs and symptoms in column 3.

Disorder	Hormone Problem	Major Signs and Symptoms
Diabetes insipidus	Antidiuretic hormone (ADH) deficiency	Polyuria
Syndrome of inappropriate antidiuretic hormone (SIADH)	Growth hormone (GH) deficiency	Growing hands and feet
Cushing's syndrome	High serum calcium	Moon face
Addison's disease	ADH excess	Labile hypertension
Graves' disease	Steroid excess	Tetany
Hypothyroidism	Deficient steroids	Muscle weakness, brittle bones
Pheochromocytoma	Epinephrine excess	Failure to grow and develop
Hyperparathyroidism	GH excess	Water retention
Short stature	Low T_3 and T_4	Weight gain and fatigue
Acromegaly	Low serum calcium	Exophthalmos
Hypoparathyroidism	High T_3 and T_4	Hypotension

CRITICAL THINKING

Read the following case studies and answer the questions.

Mr. Samuels is diagnosed with SIADH related to lung cancer. He enters the hospital for treatment of symptoms.

1. What (fluid-related) nursing diagnosis would be most appropriate for Mr. Samuels? _____

_____

2. How will you monitor Mr. Samuels' fluid balance?

_____

_____

3. Why is Mr. Samuels at risk for seizures? _____

_____

_____

_____

4. How will you reduce his risk for injury from seizures?

_____

_____

_____

5. What do you expect Mr. Samuels's urine to look like?

_____

_____

_____

6. How will Mr. Samuels's urine look after treatment is begun? _____

_____

_____

Mrs. Jorgensen is hospitalized following a motor vehicle accident in which she sustained a head injury. She develops diabetes insipidus (DI).

7. Why does head injury place Mrs. Jorgensen at risk for DI?

_____

_____

_____

8. What symptoms do diabetes insipidus and diabetes mellitus (DM) have in common? _____

_____

_____

_____

9. Will Mrs. Jorgensen's urine specific gravity be high or low? Why? _____

_____

_____

10. Will Mrs. Jorgensen's serum osmolality be high or low? Why? _____

_____

_____

11. For which (fluid-related) nursing diagnosis is Mrs. Jorgensen at risk? _____

_____

_____

12. Mrs. Jorgensen begins treatment with DDAVP (desmopressin acetate tablets). To what signs of overdose should Mrs. Jorgensen be alert?

_____

_____

_____

THYROID DISORDERS

Label each symptom with an R if it suggests hyperthyroidism or an O if it suggests hypothyroidism.

1. _____ Bradycardia
2. _____ Lethargy
3. _____ Restlessness
4. _____ Frequent stools
5. _____ Hypercholesterolemia
6. _____ Dry hair
7. _____ Tremor
8. _____ Insomnia
9. _____ Mental dullness, confusion
10. _____ Warm, diaphoretic skin
11. _____ Weight loss
12. _____ Decreased appetite

REVIEW QUESTIONS—CONTENT REVIEW

Choose the best answer unless directed otherwise.

1. Following surgery for thyroidectomy, the nurse watches carefully for which of the following signs and symptoms of tetany?
   1. Numb fingers, muscle cramps
   2. Weakness, muscle fatigue
   3. Hallucinations, delusions
   4. Dyspnea and tachycardia

2. What assessment findings should the nurse monitor to detect the onset of thyrotoxicosis in a patient with hyperthyroidism?
   1. Peripheral pulses
   2. Serum sodium
   3. Vital signs
   4. Incision site

3. Which of the following dietary recommendations will reduce the risk of kidney stones in the patient with hyperparathyroidism?
   1. Limit meat products
   2. Limit bread products
   3. Increase fluids
   4. Increase citrus fruits

4. An excess of which hormone is responsible for acromegaly?
   1. Thyroid stimulating hormone (TSH)
   2. Insulin
   3. Growth hormone (GH)
   4. Adrenocorticotropic hormone (ACTH)

5. Which of the following nursing diagnoses is most appropriate for the patient admitted in addisonian crisis?
   1. Imbalanced Nutrition: More than Body Requirements
   2. Disturbed Body Image
   3. Deficient Fluid Volume
   4. Acute Pain

REVIEW QUESTIONS—TEST PREPARATION

Choose the best answer unless directed otherwise.

6. A 42-year-old patient enters an outpatient clinic with symptoms of weight gain and fatigue. Laboratory studies are done, and a diagnosis of primary hypothyroidism is made. The patient asks why the TSH level is elevated. Which of the following is the best response by the nurse?
   1. "The thyroid makes more TSH to take the place of the deficient T_3 and T_4."
   2. "The TSH tries to directly raise the metabolic rate when there is not enough T_3 and T_4."
   3. "The pituitary makes more TSH to try to stimulate the underactive thyroid."
   4. "The extra fat cells from your weight gain make excess TSH."

7. Which of the following nursing diagnoses would be most appropriate for a patient with fatigue related to hypothyroidism?
   1. *Imbalanced Nutrition: More Than Body Requirements* related to excessive food intake
   2. *Impaired Gas Exchange* related to weight gain
   3. *Activity Intolerance* related to fatigue
   4. *Ineffective Coping* related to depression

8. A patient with hypothyroidism is started on levothyroxine (Synthroid). Which of the following statements shows that the patient understands teaching related to the new medication?
   1. "I know I should call my doctor if my heart races."
   2. "I understand that I may develop a moon-shaped face."
   3. "The sleepiness I experience when I start this medication will subside within 2 weeks."
   4. "I'll have to watch my diet to avoid further weight gain while on this medication."

9. A 26-year-old patient is hospitalized for radioactive iodine treatment for hyperthyroidism. Which of the following precautions by the nurse is appropriate?
   1. Talk with the patient only over the intercom system.
   2. Wear gloves when emptying the bedside commode.
   3. Maintain reverse isolation for 3 months.
   4. No precautions are necessary because the dose is so small.

10. The nurse needs to accomplish all the following interventions for a patient who is 24 hours post-thyroidectomy. Place the interventions in the correct order in which they should be completed.
    1. Check the surgical site dressing for signs of bleeding.
    2. Verify that the airway is patent.
    3. Assess vital signs.
    4. Administer an analgesic for postoperative pain.
    5. Teach the patient about Synthroid (levothyroxine) use after discharge.
    6. Assist with range of motion exercises of the neck.

11. The nurse develops the nursing diagnosis of *Acute Pain* related to bone demineralization for a patient with hypoparathyroidism. Which of the following goals is most appropriate?
    1. Serum calcium level will be <20mg/dL.
    2. Patient will state correct dietary restrictions.
    3. Patient will perform activities of daily living (ADLs) without injury.
    4. Patient will verbalize acceptable pain level.

12. A patient enters a clinic with possible Cushing's syndrome. Which of the following physical examination findings support this diagnosis?
    1. Weight loss, pale skin
    2. Buffalo hump, easy bruising
    3. Nausea, vomiting
    4. Polyuria, polydipsia

13. Which data is most important for the nurse to monitor in a patient with a pheochromocytoma?
    1. Vital signs
    2. Daily weights
    3. Peripheral pulses
    4. Bowel sounds

Nursing Care of Patients With Disorders of the Endocrine Pancreas

40

VOCABULARY

Fill in the blanks.

1. Glucose in the urine is called _____.

2. _____ is too much sugar in the blood.

3. _____ is too little sugar in the blood.

4. Deep, sighing respirations from diabetic acidosis are called _____ respirations.

5. Excessive hunger is called _____.

6. Excessive thirst is called _____.

7. The term used to document getting up to urinate at night is _____.

8. The time when insulin is working its hardest after injection is called its _____ action time.

9. The length of time insulin works is called its _____.

10. The Diabetes Control and Complications Trial (DCCT) found that individuals who maintain _____ control of their diabetes will have fewer long-term complications.

HYPOGLYCEMIA AND HYPERGLYCEMIA

Place an R in front of each symptom of hyperglycemia and an O in front of each symptom of hypoglycemia.

1. _____ Tremor

2. _____ Polydipsia

3. _____ Polyuria

4. _____ Lethargy

5. _____ Irritability

6. _____ Fruity breath

7. _____ Sweating

8. _____ Abdominal pain

LONG-TERM COMPLICATIONS OF DIABETES

Match the complication with its signs and symptoms.

1. _____ Retinopathy
2. _____ Neuropathy
3. _____ Hyperosmolar hyperglycemic state
4. _____ Diabetic ketoacidosis (DKA)
5. _____ Nephropathy
6. _____ Gastroparesis
7. _____ Infection

1. Ketones in the blood and urine
2. Burning pain in legs and feet
3. Fever
4. Profound hyperglycemia without ketonemia
5. Impaired vision
6. Food intolerance
7. Microalbuminuria

CRITICAL THINKING

Read the following case study and answer the questions.

Jennie is a 56-year-old overweight woman admitted to your medical unit with cellulitis of the left leg. She has a long history of diabetes mellitus; her blood sugar level is 436. She tells you that she takes insulin glargine (Lantus) 18 units every bedtime and insulin lispro (Humalog) 12 units with each meal. She also takes metformin (Glucophage) twice a day.

1. Jennie tells you that her physician wants her to keep her blood sugar level between 100 and 150 mg/dL. You know that a
   normal blood sugar level is 70 to 100. Why the discrepancy? _____
   _____
   _____
   _____

2. When you enter Jennie's room to check her 1600 vital signs, she says she has a headache. By the time you finish taking
   her blood pressure, she has developed a cold sweat. What is happening? What should you do? _____
   _____
   _____
   _____

3. At 1700, you check Jennie's blood sugar level and find that it is 80 mg/dL. What is your next step? _____
   _____
   _____
   _____

4. List three things that may have caused Jennie's blood sugar level to drop.
   _____
   _____
   _____

5. You explain to Jennie the importance of eating three meals a day on a regular schedule. She asks why. How do you explain this to her? _____
   _____
   _____
   _____

6. Jennie is discharged and follows her diet, exercise, and insulin regimen carefully. She even loses 50 lb. One year after her first admission, she is brought into the emergency department with a blood sugar level of 32. Why has her blood sugar level dropped? _____

_____

_____

7. What are two ways that metformin works? _____

_____

_____

_____

_____

8. Does Jennie have type 1 or type 2 diabetes? How do you know? _____

_____

_____

_____

REVIEW QUESTIONS—CONTENT REVIEW

Choose the best answer unless directed otherwise.

1. Which of the following is an acceptable premeal blood sugar range for most patients with diabetes?
   1. 46 to 98 mg/dL
   2. 70 to 130 mg/dL
   3. 180 to 250 mg/dL
   4. 350 to 600 mg/dL

2. Before giving insulin, the nurse always checks which test result?
   1. Recent potassium level
   2. Blood glucose level
   3. Urine ketones
   4. White blood cell count

3. At what point after injection does the peak action of insulin lispro (Humalog) occur?
   1. 30 to 90 minutes
   2. 2 to 3 hours
   3. 4 to 5 hours
   4. 8 to 12 hours

4. Which of the following are symptoms of hypoglycemia?
   1. Nausea and vomiting
   2. Glycosuria
   3. Cold sweat and tremor
   4. Polyuria and polydipsia

5. In addition to stimulating insulin production, glyburide (Micronase) has which of the following effects?
   1. Stimulates gluconeogenesis.
   2. Promotes fat breakdown.
   3. Increases tissue sensitivity to insulin.
   4. Enhances appetite.

REVIEW QUESTIONS—TEST PREPARATION

Choose the best answer unless directed otherwise.

6. A 26-year-old patient is admitted to the hospital with a new diagnosis of diabetes, a blood glucose of 680 mg/dL, and ketones in the blood and urine. Which type of diabetes should the nurse suspect?
   1. Type 1
   2. Type 2
   3. Prediabetes
   4. Gestational

7. A patient with diabetes forgot to take a daily dose of glyburide (Micronase). For which of the following symptoms should the nurse be vigilant?
   1. Cold, clammy sweat
   2. Tachycardia, nervousness, hunger
   3. Chest pain, shortness of breath
   4. Fatigue, thirst, blurred vision

8. By which routes can insulin be administered? **Select all that apply.**
   1. Oral
   2. Topical
   3. Intravenous (IV)
   4. Subcutaneous
   5. Intramuscular

9. While providing discharge instructions to a patient newly taking NPH insulin every morning, the nurse recognizes that teaching has been effective if the patient knows to observe for signs and symptoms of low blood sugar level at which of the following times?
   1. 1 hour after administration of insulin
   2. 6 to 12 hours after administration of insulin
   3. 24 to 36 hours after administration of insulin
   4. NPH insulin does not cause low blood sugar level

10. A patient with newly diagnosed diabetes asks the nurse what to take for low blood sugar. Which of the following would be most appropriate for the nurse to suggest?
    1. Raisins
    2. Cheese
    3. acetaminophen (Tylenol)
    4. Beef jerky

11. The nurse recognizes that teaching is effective if a patient with diabetes knows to use subcutaneous glucagon for an emergency episode of which of the following conditions?
    1. Hyperglycemia
    2. Ketonuria
    3. Diabetic ketoacidosis
    4. Hypoglycemia

12. A patient on an American Diabetes Association diet receives a breakfast tray and does not care for the oatmeal. Which of the following foods can the nurse substitute for a half cup of oatmeal?
    1. 4 oz of orange juice
    2. Two strips of bacon
    3. 1 oz of cheese
    4. A slice of wheat toast

Understanding the Genitourinary and Reproductive System

CHECKLIST FOR LEARNING SUCCESS

Review of Anatomy and Physiology and Aging Changes

- ❏ Female reproductive system
- ❏ Female hormones
- ❏ The menstrual cycle
- ❏ Male reproductive system
- ❏ Male hormones
- ❏ Aging changes

Major Disorders

- ❏ Breast cancer
- ❏ Menstrual disorders
- ❏ Endometriosis
- ❏ Infections
- ❏ Displacement disorders
- ❏ Fertility disorders
- ❏ Tumors of the cervix, uterus, and ovaries
- ❏ Prostatitis
- ❏ Benign prostatic hypertrophy (BPH)
- ❏ Prostate cancer
- ❏ Penile disorders
- ❏ Testicular disorders
- ❏ Erectile dysfunction
- ❏ Sexually transmitted infections (STIs)

Nursing Assessment

- ❏ History
- ❏ Breast examination
- ❏ Breast self-examination (BSE)
- ❏ Sexual function
- ❏ Testicular self-examination (TSE)

Diagnostic Tests

- ❏ Mammogram
- ❏ Biopsy
- ❏ Bone health assessment
- ❏ Hormone tests
- ❏ Pelvic examination
- ❏ Papanicolaou (Pap) smear
- ❏ Swabs and smears
- ❏ Endoscopic examinations
- ❏ Cystourethroscopy
- ❏ Digital rectal examination (DRE)
- ❏ Prostate-specific antigen (PSA)
- ❏ Fertility testing

Interventions

- ❏ Breast surgeries
- ❏ Hysterectomy
- ❏ Contraception
- ❏ Pregnancy termination
- ❏ Prostatectomy
- ❏ Transurethral resection of the prostate (TURP)
- ❏ STI prevention

Common Medications

- ❏ Antibiotics
- ❏ Hormone replacement therapy
- ❏ Oral contraceptives

41

Genitourinary and Reproductive System Function and Assessment

VOCABULARY

Complete the following sentences with the correct term from the chapter.

1. A _____ may be done to view the inside of the uterus with an endoscope.
2. During some diagnostic procedures, a body cavity is filled with carbon dioxide to make it easier for the physician to view structures. This is called _____.
3. A male patient should have a yearly _____ examination to detect prostate cancer.
4. Some men have excessive breast tissue, which is called _____.
5. If the urethral opening is on the underside of the penis, it is called _____.
6. Fluid in the scrotum is called a _____.
7. If the scrotum feels like a bag of worms when palpated, it is called a _____.
8. Another word for sexual desire is _____.
9. The beginning of menstruation in the female is called _____.
10. X-ray examination of the breasts is called _____.

ANATOMY AND PHYSIOLOGY

Label the structures of the male and female reproductive systems.

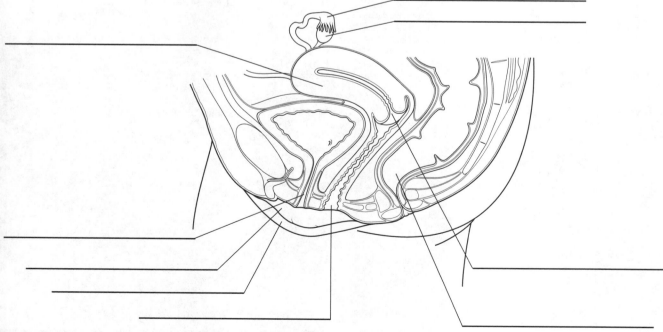

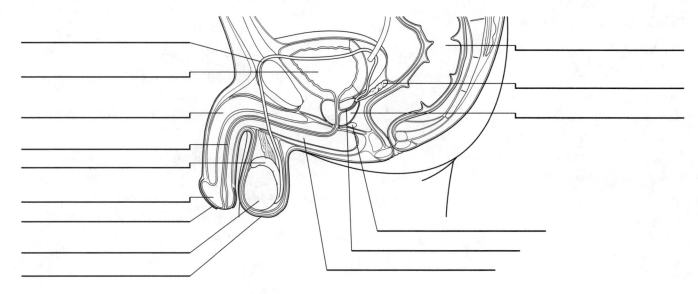

FEMALE REPRODUCTIVE STRUCTURES

Match the female reproductive structures with the correct descriptive statement.

1. _____ Fallopian tube
2. _____ Myometrium
3. _____ Bartholin's glands
4. _____ Vestibule
5. _____ Endometrium
6. _____ Ovarian follicle
7. _____ Corpus luteum

1. Site of development of an ovum
2. Becomes the maternal side of the placenta
3. Contains the urethral and vaginal openings
4. Secretes progesterone and estrogen after ovulation
5. The usual site of fertilization
6. Secrete mucus at the vaginal orifice
7. Contracts for labor and delivery

MALE REPRODUCTIVE SYSTEM

Number the following in proper sequence with respect to the pathway sperm travel from their site of origin.

_____ Ejaculatory duct
_____ Epididymis
_____ Urethra
_____ Testes
_____ Ductus deferens

DIAGNOSTIC TESTS REVIEW

Match the following tests with their descriptions.

1. _____ Cytology
2. _____ Colposcopy
3. _____ Sonography
4. _____ Computed tomographic (CT) scan
5. _____ Magnetic resonance imaging
6. _____ Digital rectal examination (DRE)

1. Endoscopic examination of the vagina
2. Examination of cells using a microscope
3. Mapping of tissues according to their densities using sound waves
4. Mapping of tissue by using radio-frequency radiation and magnetic fields
5. Screening examination for prostate disorders
6. Computer-assisted recording of very precise x-ray pictures of layers of tissue

CRITICAL THINKING

Read the scenarios and answer the following questions.

1. Mr. White comes to see his physician for a yearly checkup. As you are taking his blood pressure, he says, "I don't need that rectal examination, do I? I had prostate surgery last year." How do you respond?

   _____

   _____

   _____

   _____

2. Mrs. Bitner has just returned from having an endoscopic examination. She says, "Something went wrong, I just know it. Look at my belly. I look like I'm 9 months pregnant." How do you respond?

   _____

   _____

   _____

   _____

3. Ms. Wilson comes to the clinic and reports excessive vaginal discharge. While asking her some initial questions, you learn that she has multiple sex partners. What do you anticipate for her examination? What teaching is important? _____

   _____

   _____

   _____

4. Mr. Brown is being admitted to the hospital for complications of diabetes. While collecting initial data, you learn that although he is married, he is no longer sexually active. How do you respond? _____

   _____

   _____

   _____

REVIEW QUESTIONS—CONTENT REVIEW

Choose the best answer unless directed otherwise.

1. Which of the following male reproductive structures carries semen through the penis to the exterior?
   1. Urethra
   2. Epididymis
   3. Ductus deferens
   4. Ejaculatory duct

2. Which layer of the uterus will become the maternal portion of the placenta?
   1. Myometrium
   2. Endometrium
   3. Epimetrium
   4. Serosa

3. Which of the following descriptions best describes the position of the uterus?
   1. Superior to the bladder with the fundus most anterior
   2. Anterior to the bladder with the cervix most inferior
   3. Inferior to the bladder with the cervix most superior
   4. Posterior to the bladder with the fundus most inferior

4. Which of the following hormones stimulates the mammary glands to produce milk after pregnancy?
   1. Progesterone
   2. Estrogen
   3. Oxytocin
   4. Prolactin

5. Strong contractions of the smooth muscle of the uterus for labor and delivery are brought about by which of the following hormones?
   1. Progesterone
   2. Follicle-stimulating hormone (FSH)
   3. Oxytocin
   4. Luteinizing hormone (LH)

6. According to the American Cancer Society, how often should a 40-year-old woman have a mammogram done?
   1. Weekly
   2. Monthly
   3. Yearly
   4. Semiannually

7. When should men over age 40 have digital rectal examinations?
   1. Weekly
   2. Monthly
   3. Every other month
   4. During yearly physician visit

REVIEW QUESTIONS—TEST PREPARATION

Choose the best answer unless directed otherwise.

8. A patient being prepared for cystourethrography asks what is going to be done to him. Which is the best explanation by the nurse?
   1. "The doctor will put a tiny endoscope into your bladder."
   2. "You will have a catheter put in, then a dye will be injected and x-rays will be taken."
   3. "You will have a small needle inserted through your lower abdomen and into your bladder."
   4. "You will have an intravenous injection of dye, then x-rays will be taken as it travels through your kidneys."

9. The nurse is helping a woman prepare for a routine Pap smear. Which of the following actions should the nurse take?
   1. Give the woman an enema.
   2. Ask the woman to empty her bladder.
   3. Ask the woman to take a deep breath and hold it.
   4. Set out a suture tray and local anesthetic.

10. A nurse is teaching BSE. Which of the following positions would the nurse advise the patient to use for a portion of the exam?
    1. Supine
    2. Simm's
    3. Kneeling
    4. Fowler's

11. A woman receives notice that her screening mammogram is abnormal, and she is instructed to schedule diagnostic scans. The woman calls the office and asks the nurse, "Can you please tell me why I need more tests?" The nurse will base the response on which of the following understandings?
    1. A mammogram needs no other verification.
    2. Mammograms are unable to show lesions in breast tissue.
    3. A mammogram can show only breast cysts, not cancers.
    4. Many things can cause shadows on a mammogram besides cancer.

12. A nurse practitioner completes a wet-mount specimen on a patient with a suspected STI, then leaves the room. As the assisting LPN prepares to take the slide to the lab, the patient says, "I'm really scared that I have something serious. What do you think I should do?" Which response by the LPN is best?
    1. Sit next to the patient and say, "What frightens you the most?"
    2. Stand at the foot of the examination table and say, "There is nothing to be worried about until we get the test results."
    3. Give the patient time to verbalize concerns, then advise that she have her partner tested.
    4. Touch her lightly on the arm and say, "Let me get this slide to the lab, then I'll come back and we'll talk."

Nursing Care of Women With Reproductive System Disorders

42

VOCABULARY

Match the term with its definition.

1. _____ Imperforate	1. Bladder sags into vaginal space
2. _____ Colporrhaphy	2. Painful menstruation
3. _____ Dysmenorrhea	3. Not having expected opening
4. _____ Cryotherapy	4. Surgical repair of a part of the vagina
5. _____ Agenesis	5. Undeveloped
6. _____ Dyspareunia	6. Rectum sags into the vagina
7. _____ Cystocele	7. Painful intercourse
8. _____ Rectocele	8. Forward turning
9. _____ Anteversion	9. Removal of the ovaries
10. _____ Oophorectomy	10. Freezing of tissue

BREAST SURGERIES

Match the following breast surgery terms with their descriptions.

1. _____ Mastopexy	1. Surgery to remove a breast
2. _____ Mastectomy	2. Surgery to increase the size of the breasts
3. _____ Reduction mammoplasty	3. Surgery to decrease the size of the breasts
4. _____ Augmentation mammoplasty	4. Surgery to rebuild a breast after mastectomy
5. _____ Reconstructive mammoplasty	5. Surgery to change the position of the breasts

MENSTRUAL DISORDERS

Match the following menstrual disorders with their definitions.

1. _____ Amenorrhea	1. Difficult or painful menstruation
2. _____ Menorrhagia	2. Menses more often than every 21 days
3. _____ Dysmenorrhea	3. Passing more than 80 mL of blood per menses
4. _____ Polymenorrhea	4. Less than expected amount of menstrual bleeding
5. _____ Hypomenorrhea	5. Absence of menstrual periods for 6 months or three previous cycle lengths once cycles have been established

MASTECTOMY CARE

Circle the six errors in the following scenario and write the correct information in the space provided.

You are assigned to care for Mrs. Joseph, who is 1 day post-operative following a right radical mastectomy. You know that she is not anxious, because she had a left mastectomy a year ago and knows everything to expect. You listen to her breath sounds and find them clear, so it is not necessary to have her cough and deep breathe. You encourage her to lie on her right side to prevent bleeding. You use her right arm for blood pressures, because both arms are affected and the right one is more convenient. You also encourage her to avoid use of her right arm to prevent injury to the surgical site. You provide a balanced diet and plenty of fluids to aid in her recovery.

_____

_____

_____

_____

_____

CRITICAL THINKING

Read the following case study and answer the questions.

A 21-year-old female college student comes in to the physician's office where you work and comments with evident frustration that she has a yeast infection again. She has type 1 diabetes mellitus and takes her insulin routinely. However, she seldom tests her blood glucose level, because, she says, "I don't have time to mess with that stuff as often as I should." She comments that every time she goes home on weekends to visit her parents (a 3-hour bus trip), she develops a very uncomfortable vaginal yeast infection.

1. What factors may be contributing to her frequent yeast overgrowths? _____

_____

_____

2. What suggestions can you give her to help prevent this problem? _____

_____

_____

_____

REVIEW QUESTIONS—CONTENT REVIEW

Choose the best answer unless directed otherwise.

1. How will a douche affect a vaginal examination to determine the type of pathogen present?
   1. A douche will help clear the area for better visualization.
   2. A douche does not affect the outcome negatively or positively.
   3. Douching can wash away evidence of the pathogen, making diagnosis difficult.
   4. Douching is recommended before the examination to neutralize the pH.

2. Which of the following is a known risk factor for cervical cancer?
   1. Tight clothing
   2. A high-sodium diet
   3. Multiple sexual partners
   4. Beginning sexual activity late in life

3. Which of the following is a risk factor for development of breast cancer?
   1. Late menarche
   2. High-fat diet
   3. Early menopause
   4. Early first pregnancy

Choose the best answer unless directed otherwise.

4. Which of the following lifestyle habits are most likely to increase premenstrual syndrome symptoms? Select all that apply.
   1. Drinking alcohol
   2. Smoking
   3. Drinking coffee
   4. Eating a low-salt diet
   5. Avoiding exercise before menses

5. A nurse is teaching a patient about use of a condom with spermicide for contraception. Which statement by the patient indicates the need for further teaching?
   1. "This method will be affordable."
   2. "I am glad that barrier methods are 100% effective."
   3. "I'm glad there are fewer side effects than there are with the pill."
   4. "I know that both I and my husband will need to be diligent to use the method all the time."

6. Place the following nursing diagnoses for the woman who has just had a mastectomy for breast cancer in correct priority order.
   1. Ineffective Tissue Perfusion
   2. Risk for Ineffective Coping
   3. Ineffective Breathing Pattern
   4. Anxiety

7. Which of the following nursing interventions will help prevent swelling after a radical mastectomy with lymph node removal?
   1. Restricting all movement of the affected arm
   2. Raising the affected arm above the heart on pillows
   3. Applying warm moist heat to the arm
   4. Holding the arm close to the body with a sling

8. A patient who had a total hysterectomy 4 days ago for endometrial cancer learns that she has metastases to her lungs. When asked about her plans after discharge, she answers sharply that she "cannot plan for any future, because there isn't going to be any!" She then starts to cry. Which of the following nursing diagnoses best fits this situation?
   1. Anticipatory Grieving
   2. Disturbed Body Image
   3. Disturbed Sleep Pattern
   4. Noncompliance

9. A patient with breast cancer is being treated with tamoxifen citrate, which deprives cancer cells of the estrogen that makes them grow. This is an example of which mode of therapy?
   1. Hormonal therapy
   2. Radiation therapy
   3. Cytotoxic chemotherapy
   4. Biological response modifier therapy

10. A 38-year-old patient had a reduction mammoplasty 4 days ago. When changing her dressing, the home care nurse notes redness, swelling, and some thick yellow drainage escaping from areas of the incision line around her left nipple. Which of the following nursing interventions is appropriate?
    1. Monitor it for 24 hours, and if there is no improvement, notify the registered nurse or physician.
    2. Inform the patient that the incision is not healing properly and that she should see her physician as soon as possible.
    3. Clean the incision with normal saline and redress it, and recheck it the following day.
    4. Promptly report the situation to the registered nurse or physician and document it in the patient's chart.

43

Nursing Care of Male Patients With Genitourinary Disorders

VOCABULARY

Fill in the blanks in the following sentences with terms from the chapter.

1. When semen goes into the bladder during intercourse, it is called _____ ejaculation.

2. An erection that lasts too long is called _____.

3. _____ is the term used to describe uncircumcised foreskin that cannot be extended over the head of the penis.

4. _____ is a cottage cheese–like secretion made by the gland of the foreskin.

5. Surgical removal of the foreskin is called _____.

6. _____ is a birth condition in which one or both of the testicles have not descended into the scrotum.

7. Inflammation or infection of a testicle is called _____.

8. The correct term for male impotence is _____.

9. A _____ is varicose veins of the scrotum.

10. Surgical interruption of the vas deferens as a method of birth control is called a _____.

DISORDERS OF THE MALE REPRODUCTIVE SYSTEM

Match the disorder with its definition.

1. _____ Benign prostatic hypertrophy (BPH)
2. _____ Hydronephrosis
3. _____ Hematuria
4. _____ Peyronie's disease
5. _____ Priapism
6. _____ Epididymitis
7. _____ Infertility
8. _____ Orchitis
9. _____ Dysuria
10. _____ Reflux

1. Blood in the urine
2. Curved penis
3. Noncancerous overgrowth of prostate tissue
4. Inability to reproduce
5. Distention of kidney with retained urine
6. Inflammation of the testicles
7. Inflammation or infection of the tube where sperm matures
8. Painful or difficult urination
9. Backward flow of urine
10. Prolonged erection

ERECTILE DYSFUNCTION REVIEW

Unscramble the following causes of erectile dysfunction.

1. aeiioctdmn _____

2. sssrte _____

3. eeiophysnntr _____

4. PRUT _____

5. threa flraeiu _____

6. tiellpum lersssoic _____

CRITICAL THINKING

Read the following case study and answer the questions.

Mr. Washington is a 62-year-old retired teacher who comes to the urgent care center reporting that he "can't pass water."

1. What initial questions do you ask to further assess Mr. Washington's problem? _____

   _____

   _____

2. What do you think is happening?

   _____

   _____

   _____

   _____

3. What care do you anticipate as the physician examines him? _____

   _____

   _____

4. What can result if the problem continues untreated?

   _____

   _____

   _____

Mr. Washington is transferred to the local hospital, where BPH is confirmed. He is scheduled for a transurethral resection of the prostate (TURP). He asks the nurse, "What's a TURP?"

5. How can the nurse explain a TURP to Mr. Washington?

   _____

   _____

   _____

6. After surgery, Mr. Washington has a three-way Foley catheter. What is the purpose of this type of catheter? How should the nurse total intake and output (I&O) at the end of the shift? _____

   _____

   _____

   _____

7. Bladder spasms are common after TURP. How will the nurse know if this is happening? What interventions will help? _____

   _____

   _____

8. Mr. Washington is discharged. The next day he calls the nursing unit and says in a panicky voice, "I just wet my pants! I can't hold my urine! This is worse than not being able to go at all!" How should the nurse respond? What can Mr. Washington do? _____

   _____

   _____

REVIEW QUESTIONS—CONTENT REVIEW

Choose the best answer unless directed otherwise.

1. Which of the following nursing actions is most appropriate when doing perineal care on an uncircumcised male patient?
   1. Leave the foreskin retracted so air can keep the area dry.
   2. Do not retract the foreskin during washing.
   3. Replace the foreskin over the head of the penis after washing.
   4. Use alcohol and a cotton swab to clean under the foreskin.

2. What should be included when teaching young men to detect testicular cancer early?
   1. Monthly testicular self-examination (TSE)
   2. Yearly digital rectal examination (DRE)
   3. Annual physician examination
   4. Annual ultrasonography

REVIEW QUESTIONS—TEST PREPARATION

Choose the best answer unless directed otherwise.

3. The nurse completes a nursing history on a patient admitted for a TURP. Which symptoms of BPH does the nurse expect the patient to report? **Select all answers that apply.**
   1. A feeling of incomplete bladder emptying after voiding
   2. Difficulty maintaining an erection
   3. Difficulty urinating
   4. Grossly bloody urine
   5. Pain in the lower back that radiates to the hips during urination
   6. Nocturia

4. A patient tells his nurse that he has delayed having a TURP because he is afraid it will affect his sexual function. Which response by the nurse is most appropriate?
   1. "Don't worry about sterility; sperm production is not affected by this surgery."
   2. "Would you like some information about implants used for impotence?"
   3. "This type of surgery rarely affects the ability to have an erection or ejaculation."
   4. "There are many methods of sexual expression that are alternatives to sexual intercourse."

5. A patient returns from surgery following a TURP with a three-way Foley catheter and continuous bladder irrigation. Postoperative orders include meperidine (Demerol) 75 mg IM every three hours (q3h) as needed for pain, belladonna and opium (B&O) suppository q4h as needed, and strict I&O. The patient reports painful bladder spasms, and the nurse observes blood-tinged urine on the sheets. Which action should the nurse take first?
   1. Give the Demerol.
   2. Give the B&O suppository.
   3. Warm the irrigation solution to body temperature.
   4. Notify the physician stat.

6. A patient who has just had a TURP asks his nurse to explain why he has to have the bladder irrigation because it seems to increase his pain. Which of the following explanations by the nurse is best?
   1. "The bladder irrigation is needed to stop the bleeding in the bladder."
   2. "Antibiotics are being administered into the bladder to prevent infection."
   3. "The irrigation is needed to keep the catheter from becoming occluded by blood clots."
   4. "Normal production of urine is maintained with the irrigations until healing can occur."

7. A post-TURP patient experiences dribbling following removal of his catheter. Which action should the nurse take?
   1. Have him restrict fluid intake to 1000 mL/day.
   2. Teach him to perform Kegel's exercises 10 to 20 times per hour.
   3. Reinsert the Foley catheter until he regains urinary control.
   4. Reassure him that incontinence never lasts more than a few days.

8. A 36-year-old man is scheduled for a unilateral orchiectomy for treatment of testicular cancer. He is withdrawn and does not interact with the nurse. Which action is most appropriate?
   1. Identify the problem with a nursing diagnosis of *Impaired Communication* related to the diagnosis of cancer.
   2. Set a patient outcome that the patient will verbalize his concerns about his diagnosis.
   3. Ask the patient whether he is worried about future sexual functioning.
   4. Say, "You seem quiet. Are you feeling concerned about your diagnosis or treatment?"

9. A 28-year-old man is diagnosed with acute epididymitis. For which of the following symptoms should the nurse assess?
   1. Burning and pain on urination
   2. Severe tenderness and swelling in the scrotum
   3. Foul-smelling ejaculate and severe scrotal swelling
   4. Foul-smelling urine and pain on urination

10. A man with a history of diabetes and chronic lung disease is admitted to the hospital with prostate cancer. He has all the following symptoms. Which should the nurse address first?
    1. Fever of 101°F (38.3°C)
    2. Respiratory rate of 36 per minute
    3. Difficulty urinating
    4. Painful legs and feet

11. The nurse is providing care for a patient scheduled for a vasectomy. Which of the following statements indicates further teaching is necessary?
    1. "I will need to have my testosterone levels checked periodically to ensure the success of the surgery."
    2. "Another method of birth control should be used for the next three months."
    3. "The amount and color of my ejaculate should be the same as before surgery."
    4. "I'll have to bring a sample of semen back for evaluation after the surgery."

Nursing Care of Patients With Sexually Transmitted Infections

44

VOCABULARY

Match the term with its definition.

1. _____ Condylomatous
2. _____ Gumma
3. _____ Chancre
4. _____ Cytotoxic
5. _____ Herpetic
6. _____ Puerperal

1. Relating to herpes
2. Rubbery tumor
3. Red ulcer from syphilis
4. Wartlike
5. Poison to cells
6. Time following childbirth

INFLAMMATORY DISORDERS

Match the following inflammation words with their definitions.

1. _____ Proctitis
2. _____ Urethritis
3. _____ Cervicitis
4. _____ Endometritis
5. _____ Conjunctivitis

1. Inflammation of the rectum and anus
2. Inflammation of the cervix
3. Inflammation of the urethra
4. Inflammation of parts of the eye
5. Inflammation of the lining of the uterus

BARRIER METHODS FOR SAFER SEX

List the teaching that should accompany each of the following barriers against sexually transmitted infections (STIs).

1. Male condoms _____

_____

2. Female condoms _____

_____

_____

_____

3. Diaphragms _____

_____

_____

4. Rubber gloves _____
_____
_____
_____

5. Double condoms _____
_____
_____
_____

CRITICAL THINKING

Read the following case study and answer the questions.

James, 32 years old, arrives at an outpatient clinic requesting STI testing for him and his fiancée. You learn that he met his fiancée through an international dating agency and that she has come here to marry him. She does not speak English. He asks you to give him the paperwork for both of them to get the blood test for STIs—just to make sure they don't have anything contagious. He seems in a hurry and asks if they can have their blood drawn first and then he could come back in an hour or two and see the doctor for the results for both of them.

1. What misunderstandings does James have about STI diagnosis? _____
_____
_____

2. Legally and ethically, does James have a right to be told his fiancée's test results? _____
_____
_____
_____

3. What procedures should occur before any testing is done? _____
_____
_____
_____

4. Is James likely to get his answer about whether either he or his fiancée has a contagious STI today? _____
_____
_____
_____
_____

REVIEW QUESTIONS—CONTENT REVIEW

Choose the best answer unless directed otherwise.

1. Which STI is associated with gummas?
   1. Gonorrhea
   2. Herpes simplex
   3. Trichomoniasis
   4. Syphilis

2. Which virus causes genital warts?
   1. Cytomegalovirus
   2. Herpes simplex virus type II
   3. Human papillomavirus
   4. Human immunodeficiency virus

REVIEW QUESTIONS—TEST PREPARATION

Choose the best answer unless directed otherwise.

3. A 36-year-old woman who has had no prenatal care comes into the hospital in active labor for her fourth child. She has vesicles evident on her perineum. Which of the following nursing actions are appropriate to protect the unborn baby and the staff? **Select all that apply.**
   1. Maintain standard precautions.
   2. Reprimand the mother for putting her baby at risk for herpes.
   3. Prepare for the possibility that the baby may be delivered by cesarean section.
   4. Notify the obstetrician or nurse midwife about the vesicles as soon as possible.
   5. Apply antibiotic ointment to the vesicles.
   6. Place the mother in reverse isolation.

4. A 23-year-old woman is seen at an outpatient clinic for a routine Papanicolaou (Pap) smear. When questioned, she states she is deciding whether to engage in sexual activity with a man she is just getting to know. She asks how she can tell if he has an STI. Which response by the nurse is best?
   1. "If the man appears clean and has been conscientious about using condoms, he is likely infection free."
   2. "Look carefully for signs of lesions before engaging in sexual activity."
   3. "Be sure to use either a male or female condom to protect against possible transmission of infection."
   4. "An examination by a physician with diagnostic testing is the only way to know if he is infection free."

5. A college student goes to the college clinic and asks the best way to avoid contracting an STI. The nurse provides the clinic's standard STI teaching. Which statement by the student indicates the need for additional instruction?
   1. "There is no guarantee that I won't contract an STI if I choose to be sexually active."
   2. "Abstinence is the only sure way to avoid an STI."
   3. "If I use a condom with spermicide, I will be safer than if I don't use one."
   4. "If I question my partner about past sexual encounters, I can avoid STIs."

6. While bathing an 82-year-old man hospitalized with pneumonia, a nurse notes an ulcerated area on his penis. What action should the nurse take first?
   1. Report the ulcer to the admitting care provider.
   2. Teach the man about STI prevention.
   3. Ask the man if he has a history of syphilis.
   4. Clean the ulcer; reporting is not necessary because an STI is unlikely in a man this age.

7. A 16-year-old girl is diagnosed with genital herpes. She has vesicles on her genitals and urethritis. She is tearful as she asks what she can do to prevent complications of the disease. On the basis of the data provided, which nursing diagnosis is appropriate for her plan of care?
   1. Risk for Infection
   2. Health-Seeking Behaviors
   3. Pain
   4. Ineffective Sexuality Pattern

8. A patient has cloudy penile discharge. For which additional symptoms of urethritis should the nurse assess?
   1. Throat or rectal infection
   2. Chancres or vesicles on the genitals
   3. Painful and frequent urination
   4. Oliguria and flank pain

9. A woman with pelvic inflammatory disease says she has lower abdominal pain. Which action should the nurse take first?
   1. Have her rate her pain on a 0 to 10 scale.
   2. Administer antibiotics as ordered.
   3. Administer an analgesic as ordered.
   4. Teach the patient about causes and prevention of STIs.

10. A nurse needs to administer an intramuscular injection of 2.4 million units of penicillin G. It is supplied in a vial of 5,000,000 units of powder for injection. Instructions state to dilute with 8 mL of sterile water. How many mL should the nurse draw up? _____

11. The nurse receives a phone call from a client who reports engaging in recent sexual activity with a partner who just informed her that he has herpes. Which of the following statements by the nurse is best?
   1. "How long has your partner had herpes?"
   2. "Did you notice any rash or other lesions on his face or genitalia?"
   3. "You need to use a diaphragm if you engage in sexual intercourse with him again."
   4. "If you notice flulike symptoms, symptoms of a bladder infection, or vaginal drainage within the next two weeks you need to be seen right away."

unit TWELVE

Understanding the Musculoskeletal System

CHECKLIST FOR LEARNING SUCCESS

Review of Anatomy and Physiology and Aging Changes	Major Disorders	Nursing Assessment	Diagnostic Tests	Interventions	Common Medications
❑ Skeletal system	❑ Osteoarthritis	❑ History	❑ Alkaline phosphatase	❑ Amputation	❑ Allopurinol (Zyloprim)
❑ Muscular system	❑ Rheumatoid arthritis	❑ Medications	❑ Erythrocyte sedimentation rate	❑ Prosthesis	❑ Analgesics
❑ Aging effects	❑ Gout	❑ Vital signs		❑ Casts	❑ Anticoagulants
	❑ Carpal tunnel syndrome	❑ Physical examination	❑ Serum calcium/phosphorus/ uric acid	❑ Closed reduction	❑ Antirheumatic drugs
	❑ Fractures	❑ Deformities/limb length	❑ Creatinine kinase	❑ Diet therapy	❑ Bisphosphonates
	❑ Complications of fractures	❑ Crepitation	❑ Myoglobin	❑ External fixation	❑ Calcitonin (Calcimar)
	❑ Rhabdomyolysis	❑ Swelling	❑ Rheumatoid factor	❑ Heat and cold	❑ Corticosteroids
	❑ Osteomyelitis	❑ Range of motion	❑ Arthrocentesis	❑ Open reduction/ internal fixation	❑ Cox-2 selective inhibitors
	❑ Osteoporosis	❑ Muscle strength	❑ Arthrography	❑ Rest, ice, compression, elevation	❑ Muscle relaxants
	❑ Paget's disease	❑ Pain	❑ Arthroscopy		❑ Nonsteroidal anti-inflammatory drugs (NSAIDs)
	❑ Bone cancer	❑ Neurovascular checks	❑ Bone scan	❑ Total joint replacement	❑ Raloxifene (Evista)
			❑ Electromyography (EMG)	❑ Traction	
			❑ Magnetic resonance imaging (MRI)		
			❑ Myelogram		
			❑ X-rays		
			❑ Dual energy x-ray absorptiometry		

45

Musculoskeletal Function and Assessment

STRUCTURE OF NEUROMUSCULAR JUNCTION AND SARCOMERES

Label the structures from the following word list.

Acetylcholine receptors
Motor Neuron
Myofilaments
Sarcolemma
Sarcomere

Sarcoplasmic reticulum
Synaptic cleft
T Tubules
Vesicle of acetylcholine

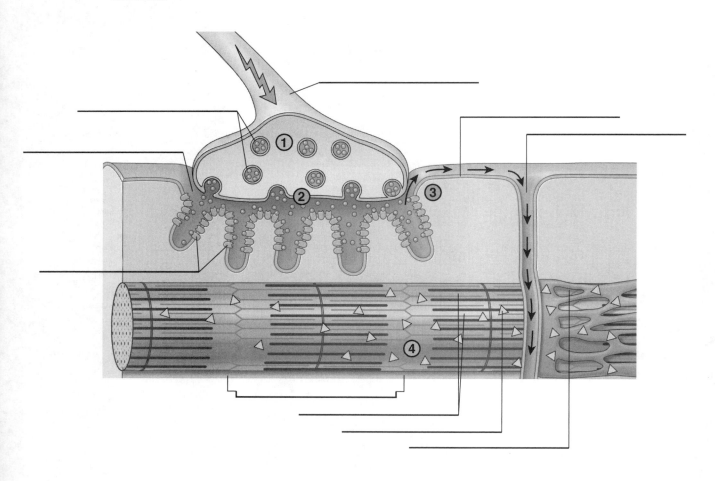

NEUROMUSCULAR JUNCTION

Match each part of the neuromuscular junction with the proper descriptions. Each part will have two correct answers.

1. _____ Synapse
2. _____ Axon terminal
3. _____ Sarcolemma

1. Contains the transmitter acetylcholine
2. The cell membrane of the muscle fiber
3. The space between the muscle fiber and the motor neuron
4. Has receptors for acetylcholine
5. An impulse is transmitted by the diffusion of acetylcholine
6. The end of the motor neuron

SYNOVIAL JOINTS

Match each part of a synovial joint with the correct function.

1. _____ Articular cartilage
2. _____ Joint capsule
3. _____ Synovial membrane
4. _____ Synovial fluid
5. _____ Bursae

1. Lines the joint capsule and secretes synovial fluid
2. Prevents friction within the joint cavity
3. Encloses the joint similar to a sleeve
4. Permit tendons to slide easily across a joint
5. Provides a smooth surface on the joint surfaces of bones

VOCABULARY

Match the word on the left with its definition on the right.

1. _____ Symphysis
2. _____ Ball and socket
3. _____ Hinge
4. _____ Condyloid
5. _____ Pivot
6. _____ Gliding
7. _____ Saddle
8. _____ Bursa
9. _____ Crepitation
10. _____ Synovitis

1. Movement in all planes
2. Rotation
3. Disk of fibrous cartilage between bones
4. Movement in one plane
5. Hinge with some lateral movement
6. Side-to-side movement
7. Small sacs of synovial fluid between joints and tendons
8. Movement in several planes
9. Swollen synovial tissue within the joint
10. Grating sound as joint or bone moves

DIAGNOSTIC TESTS

Match each diagnostic test to its appropriate description.

1. _____ X-ray
2. _____ Arthrogram
3. _____ MRI
4. _____ Arthroscopy
5. _____ Arthrocentesis
6. _____ Bone scan
7. _____ Alkaline phosphatase
8. _____ Calcium
9. _____ Phosphorus
10. _____ Erythrocyte sedimentation rate
11. _____ Uric acid
12. _____ Dual energy x-ray absorptiometry (DEXA)

1. Dye required to view joint structures: tendons, ligaments, cartilage
2. Radio waves and magnetic field view of soft tissue
3. Bones show up as white areas
4. Insertion of a needle into a joint space to remove fluid, obtain a specimen, or instill medication
5. An endoscopy of joints with local or general anesthesia
6. Serum level of enzyme that is made by osteoblasts to mineralize bone
7. After injection, a radioisotope is taken up by bone and 2 hours later a camera scans the body front and back
8. Serum level of substance stored in bone that makes bone rigid

9. Serum test for inflammation
10. Serum level of substance that mineralizes bones and teeth
11. Serum level for end product of purine metabolism
12. Special x-ray used to evaluate bone density

CRITICAL THINKING

Read the following case study and answer the questions.

Mr. John Allen, age 45, was in an automobile accident and comes to the emergency department with a fractured femur.

1. What information should the nurse include in Mr. Allen's history?

_____

_____

2. What areas should Mr. Allen's physical examination focus on first? _____

_____

_____

3. What tests can the nurse anticipate will be done on Mr. Allen? _____

_____

_____

4. What types of teaching should the nurse do?

_____

_____

_____

REVIEW QUESTIONS—CONTENT REVIEW

Choose the best answer unless directed otherwise.

1. Absorbing shock between adjacent vertebrae is the function of disks made of which of the following?
   1. Smooth muscle
   2. Synovial fluid
   3. Fibrous cartilage
   4. Adipose tissue

2. Which of the following is the transmitter at neuromuscular junctions?
   1. Sodium ions
   2. Acetylcholine
   3. A nerve impulse
   4. Cholinesterase

3. Muscles are attached to bones by which of the following?
   1. Tendons
   2. Ligaments
   3. Fascia
   4. Other muscles

4. Which of the following is the part of the brain that initiates muscle contraction?
   1. Parietal lobe
   2. Cerebellum
   3. Frontal lobe
   4. Temporal lobe

5. Which of the following organ systems is not considered directly necessary for muscle contraction?
   1. Circulatory system
   2. Digestive system
   3. Respiratory system
   4. Nervous system

6. Which of the following is the function of synovial fluid in joints?
   1. Exchange nutrients
   2. Prevent friction
   3. Absorb water
   4. Wear away rough surfaces

REVIEW QUESTIONS—TEST PREPARATION

Choose the best answer unless directed otherwise.

7. The nurse is inspecting the knee of a patient who reports pain and stiffness in it. As the patient moves the knee the nurse hears a grating sound. The nurse documents the grating sound as which of the following?
   1. Friction rub
   2. Crepitation
   3. Effusion
   4. Subcutaneous emphysema

8. The nurse is caring for a patient who reports knee pain. When the nurse observes a joint that has a grating sound with movement, which of the following actions should the nurse take next?
   1. Adduct the extremity.
   2. Flex the joint.
   3. Avoid joint movement.
   4. Abduct the extremity.

9. The nurse is gathering functional data on a patient with rheumatoid arthritis. Which of the following areas would the nurse include in the assessment?
   1. Response to treatment
   2. Ability to prepare food
   3. Appearance of joints
   4. Lung sounds

10. Following a patient's bone biopsy, the nurse inspects the biopsy site. The nurse is monitoring for which of the following complications that may occur immediately following a biopsy?
    1. Joint dislocation
    2. Crackles
    3. Infection
    4. Hematoma formation

11. The nurse is caring for a patient after a biopsy. The nurse understands that increased pain that is unresponsive to analgesic medication in a patient who has had a biopsy may indicate which of the following biopsy complications?
    1. Bleeding in soft tissue
    2. A low pain tolerance
    3. An allergic reaction
    4. Inadequate analgesic dose

46

Nursing Care of Patients With Musculoskeletal and Connective Tissue Disorders

VOCABULARY

Fill in the blank with the word that is formed by the word building.

1. _____ arthro—joint + itis—inflammation
2. _____ arthro—joint + plasty—creation of
3. _____ synovia—synovial fluid or tissue + itis—inflammation
4. _____ arthro—joint + centesis—puncture of a cavity
5. _____ hyper—excessive + uric—uric acid + emia—in blood
6. _____ vascul—blood vessel + itis—inflammation
7. _____ a—without + vascular—blood + necrosis—death
8. _____ re—again + plant—to plant + tion—process
9. _____ hemi—half + pelv—pelvis + ectomy—removal of
10. _____ fascia—fibrous tissue + otomy—opening into
11. _____ osteo—bone + myel—bone marrow + itis—inflammation
12. _____ osteo—bone + sarco—flesh + oma—tumor

FRACTURES

Match the type of fracture with its definition.

1. _____ More than two fragments that appear to float
2. _____ At right angle to bone
3. _____ Splintered and bent, occurring mainly in children
4. _____ More than two fragments driven into each other
5. _____ Extends into articular surface
6. _____ Runs along axis of bone
7. _____ Oblique fracture line
8. _____ Spontaneous fracture from bone disease
9. _____ Fracture spirals around shaft of bone
10. _____ From repeated stress (jogging)

1. Transverse
2. Stress
3. Spiral
4. Pathological
5. Oblique
6. Longitudinal
7. Interarticular
8. Impacted
9. Greenstick
10. Comminuted

PROSTHESIS CARE EDUCATION

Indicate whether the statement is true or false, and correct false statements.

1. _____ Replace shoes when they wear out with new ones of a different height and type.

2. _____ Clean the prosthesis socket with alcohol and water, and dry it completely.

3. _____ Replace worn inserts and liners when they become too soiled to clean adequately.

4. _____ Use garters to keep socks or stockings in place.

5. _____ Oil the mechanical parts as instructed by the physician.

HEALTH PROMOTION FOR PATIENTS WITH GOUT

Fill in the blanks.

1. Avoid high _____ foods, such as organ meats, shellfish, and oily fish such as _____.

2. _____ alcohol.

3. Drink plenty of _____, especially water.

4. Avoid all forms of _____ and drugs containing _____.

5. _____ diuretics.

6. Avoid excessive physical or emotional _____.

CRITICAL THINKING

Complete the nursing care plan for the nursing diagnosis Impaired Physical Mobility for a patient with a hip replacement.

NURSING DIAGNOSIS
Impaired Physical Mobility related to hip precautions and surgical pain

Interventions	Rationale	Evaluation
_____ _____ _____	Activity is restricted due to hip precautions and weight-bearing limitations.	_____ _____ _____
Place overhead frame and trapeze on bed; teach patient how to use it.	_____ _____ _____	Does patient use over-bed frame and trapeze for movement?
Monitor the patient for and take measures to prevent complications of immobility: _____ _____ _____ _____ _____ _____	_____ _____	Is the patient free from complications of immobility?

REVIEW QUESTIONS—CONTENT REVIEW

Choose the best answer unless directed otherwise.

1. Which of the following is the recommended protocol for caring for a severed body part that may be replanted?
   1. Cover it with a warm dry towel.
   2. Wrap it in a clean moist cloth.
   3. Place it directly in ice.
   4. Wrap it in a dry sterile dressing.

2. Which of these laboratory values should the nurse monitor for a patient with gout?
   1. Blood urea nitrogen
   2. Creatinine
   3. Uric acid
   4. Cholesterol

REVIEW QUESTIONS—TEST PREPARATION

Choose the best answer unless directed otherwise.

3. A patient is in skin traction using a foam boot with Velcro® fasteners for a fractured hip. The nurse would document this type of skin traction as which of the following?
   1. Gardner's tongs
   2. Buck's traction
   3. Crutchfield's tongs
   4. Steinmann's pin

4. A patient sustains a closed fracture of the right tibia and is placed in a long-leg plaster cast, which is still damp. Which of the following methods should the nurse use to move the cast without causing complications?
   1. Have the patient move own leg.
   2. Palm the cast to move it.
   3. Use fingertips to grasp cast.
   4. Avoid moving the cast until it is dry.

5. A patient is being treated with gold therapy for rheumatoid arthritis. Which of the following interventions is essential when gold therapy is started? **Select all that apply.**
   1. Removing all metal objects patient is wearing
   2. Assessing allergies to iodine
   3. Giving a test dose of gold
   4. Planning a biweekly dosing schedule
   5. Monitoring the patient after the injection
   6. Teaching the patient to perform daily weights

6. The nurse is caring for a patient who has a fractured ankle that is in a cast. The patient has morphine 10 to 15 mg intramuscularly ordered every 3 to 4 hours. The patient received morphine 10 mg 2 hours and 45 minutes ago and is rating the pain at 10+ and moans that the leg hurts. The patient has good capillary refill. Which of the following actions is most appropriate for the nurse to take next?
   1. Apply ice to the cast.
   2. Notify the physician immediately.
   3. Remove the pillow under the cast.
   4. Prepare morphine 15 mg for administration.

7. The nurse turns a 2-day postoperative patient with a right total hip replacement using three pillows between the legs. The nurse later returns and finds the patient lying supine with legs crossed. Which of the following should the nurse monitor to determine whether a complication has developed?
   1. The right knee for crepitation
   2. The left leg for internal rotation
   3. The left leg for loss of function
   4. The right leg for shortening

8. Discharge teaching for patients who have gout includes diet teaching. Patients will require additional teaching if they say they will be eating which one of the following?
   1. Cod
   2. Chicken
   3. Eggs
   4. Liver

9. Which of the following medications should a patient with gout be encouraged to avoid to prevent a gout attack?
   1. Aspirin
   2. Tylenol
   3. Nonsteroidal anti-inflammatory drugs
   4. Narcotics

10. The nurse is reviewing an erythrocyte sedimentation rate (ESR) for a patient. Which of the following does the nurse understand is the purpose of an ESR test?
    1. To identify the number of red blood cells the patient has
    2. To determine sedimentation found in red blood cells
    3. To identify the presence of systemic inflammation
    4. To diagnose various types of arthritis

11. A patient asks why a test dose of gold therapy is necessary. Which of the following is the most appropriate response by the nurse?
    1. "To avoid waste of expensive gold."
    2. "To determine the necessary dose."
    3. "To determine the therapeutic response."
    4. "To assess for an allergic reaction."

12. Which of the following symptoms would the nurse most likely be told was the first symptom that caused a patient with rheumatoid arthritis to seek health care?
    1. Cold intolerance
    2. Stiff, sore joints
    3. Shortness of breath
    4. Crepitation

unit THIRTEEN

Understanding the Neurologic System

CHECKLIST FOR LEARNING SUCCESS

Review of Anatomy and Physiology and Aging Changes	Major Disorders	Nursing Assessment	Diagnostic Tests	Interventions	Common Medications
❑ Central nervous system (CNS) structure and function ❑ Peripheral nervous system (PNS) ❑ Cranial nerves ❑ Spinal nerves ❑ Sympathetic ❑ Parasympathetic ❑ Aging changes	❑ CNS infections ❑ Increased intracranial pressure (ICP) ❑ Headaches ❑ Seizures ❑ Traumatic brain injury (TBI) ❑ Hematomas ❑ Brain tumors ❑ Herniated disk ❑ Spinal cord injury ❑ Parkinson's disease ❑ Alzheimer's disease ❑ Transient ischemic attack (TIA) ❑ Stroke—hemorrhagic, ischemic ❑ Multiple sclerosis ❑ Myasthenia gravis ❑ Amyotrophic lateral sclerosis (ALS) ❑ Guillain-Barré syndrome ❑ Postpolio syndrome ❑ Cranial nerve disorders	❑ Health history ❑ Level of consciousness (LOC; Glasgow and FOUR Score coma scales) ❑ Mental status ❑ Eyes ❑ Muscle function ❑ Cranial nerves ❑ ICP	❑ Lumbar puncture ❑ Computed tomographic (CT) scan ❑ Magnetic resonance imaging (MRI) ❑ Angiogram ❑ Myelogram ❑ Electroencephalogram (EEG)	❑ Positioning ❑ Interventions for swallowing ❑ Activities of daily living (ADLs) ❑ Communication ❑ Nutrition ❑ Rehabilitation ❑ Interventions for increased ICP ❑ Interventions for seizures ❑ Interventions for chronic confusion	❑ Anticoagulants ❑ Thrombolytics ❑ Corticosteroids ❑ Platelet aggregation inhibitors ❑ Diuretics ❑ Anticonvulsants

47

Neurologic System Function, Assessment, and Therapeutic Measures

VOCABULARY

Fill in the blank with the correct term.

1. Difficulty swallowing is called _____.
2. An _____ is a test that uses scalp electrodes to evaluate brain activity.
3. A patient might say his leg feels like it is asleep to describe _____.
4. Abnormal flexion posturing when eliciting best motor response is called _____ posturing.
5. Abnormal extension posturing when eliciting best motor response is called _____ posturing.
6. _____ is the term that describes unequal pupils.
7. Involuntary eye movement is called _____.
8. Permanent muscle contractions are called _____.
9. Difficulty speaking because of muscle dysfunction is called _____.
10. Patients who have difficulty speaking after a stroke are experiencing _____.

DIAGNOSTIC TESTS

Describe the procedure and nursing care before and after each of the following diagnostic tests used for neurological diagnoses. (See DavisPlus for complete descriptions.)

1. Myelogram _____

   _____

   _____

2. EEG _____

   _____

   _____

3. Lumbar puncture _____

   _____

   _____

4. MRI _____

   _____

   _____

5. CT scan _____
_____
_____

ANATOMY
Label the parts of the cerebrum.

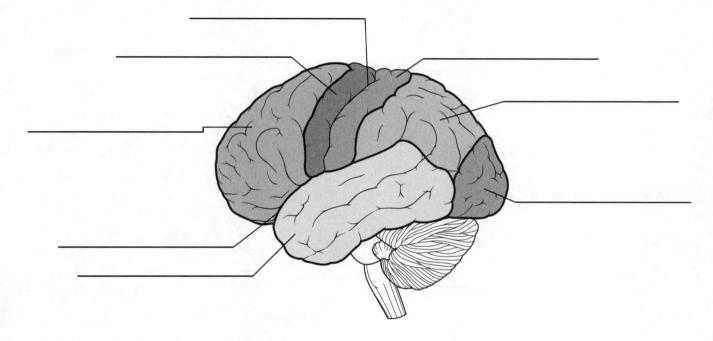

Label the parts of the neuron.

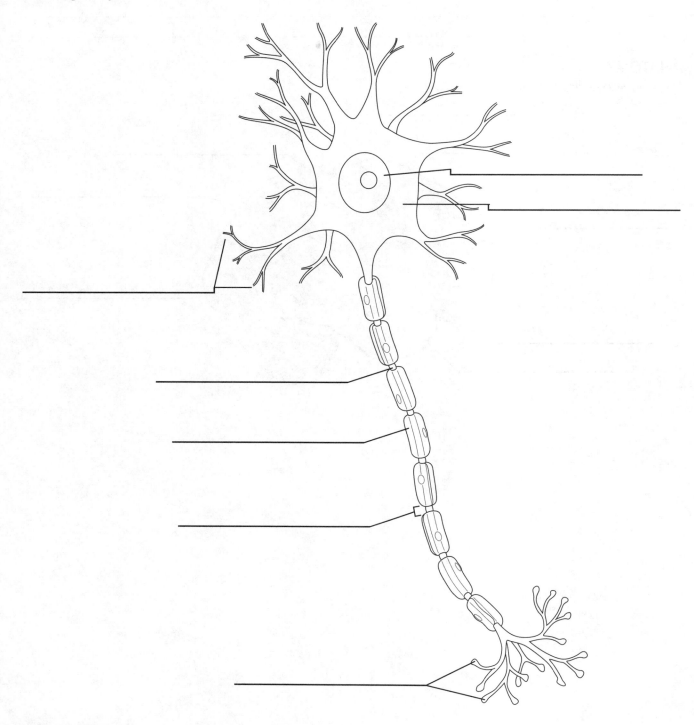

ANATOMY REVIEW

Match the part of the brain with the function it controls.

1. _____ Cerebrum

2. _____ Medulla oblongata

3. _____ Occipital lobe

4. _____ Cerebellum

5. _____ Temporal lobe

1. Vision center

2. Speech

3. Equilibrium and coordination

4. Respiratory center

5. Information storage

ASSESSMENT OF CRANIAL NERVES

Match the following assessment tools with the nerve to be tested.

1. _____ Cotton ball
2. _____ Snellen chart
3. _____ Use of hands to check neck/shoulder strength
4. _____ Tuning fork or whisper
5. _____ Tongue blade and cotton swab

1. Vestibulocochlear (VIII)
2. Accessory (XI)
3. Trigeminal (V)
4. Optic (II)
5. Vagus (X)

CRITICAL THINKING

Read the following case study and answer the following questions.

Mrs. Pickett is admitted to the nursing home where you work as a nurse. She had a stroke 2 weeks ago and is not strong enough to go to a rehabilitation facility. She has left-sided weakness. You collect admitting data to help determine her plan of care.

1. Mrs. Pickett tells you she needs to get up to go to the bathroom. What are some things you can do to determine if she is able to do this? _____
   _____
   _____
   _____

2. Mrs. Pickett's first meal is served. What can you do to determine her ability to eat safely?
   _____
   _____
   _____

3. Mrs. Pickett says, "Will you go to the kitchen and get me one of those cookies I like?" How do you determine whether she is confused? _____
   _____
   _____
   _____

4. Mrs. Pickett is weak on her left side. Why do you think her blood pressure will be more accurate in her right arm?
   _____
   _____
   _____

REVIEW QUESTIONS—CONTENT REVIEW

Choose the best answer unless directed otherwise.

1. Which of the following parts of a neuron transmits impulses away from the cell body?
   1. Dendrite
   2. Axon
   3. Neurolemma
   4. Synapse

2. Which type of neuron transmits impulses from the CNS to the muscles and glands?
   1. Afferent
   2. Efferent

3. Which part of the brain controls breathing?
   1. Medulla
   2. Cerebellum
   3. Cerebrum
   4. Thalamus

4. When a neurologist asks a patient to smile, which cranial nerve is being tested?
   1. II optic
   2. VII facial
   3. X vagus
   4. XI accessory

5. The neurologist tests the fourth (trochlear) and sixth (abducens) cranial nerves together by having a patient do which of the following?
   1. Turn his head to the right and left.
   2. Identify whispering in his ears.
   3. Say "ahhh."
   4. Follow a finger with the eyes.

6. Which of the following responses indicates sympathetic nervous system activation?
   1. Tachycardia, dilated pupils
   2. Increased peristalsis, abdominal cramping
   3. Hypoglycemia, headache
   4. Pupil constriction, bronchoconstriction

7. Which neurotransmitter mediates the sympathetic response?
   1. Acetylcholine
   2. Prostaglandin
   3. Norepinephrine
   4. Serotonin

REVIEW QUESTIONS—TEST PREPARATION

Choose the best answer unless directed otherwise.

8. Which of the following actions are controlled by nerves exiting from the cervical portion of the spinal cord? **Select all that apply.**
   1. Blinking
   2. Writing
   3. Sticking out the tongue
   4. Nodding
   5. Urinating
   6. Homans' sign

9. The nurse is assisting a patient to prepare for a lumbar puncture. Which of the following actions should the nurse take first?
   1. Administer enemas until clear.
   2. Remove all metal jewelry.
   3. Position the patient on his or her side.
   4. Remove the patient's dentures.

10. When caring for a patient who has just undergone a lumbar puncture, which of the following nursing actions takes the highest priority?
    1. Have the patient lie flat for 6 to 8 hours.
    2. Keep the patient nil per os (NPO) for 4 hours.
    3. Monitor the patient's pedal pulses every four hours.
    4. Encourage the patient to deep breathe and cough.

11. The nurse knows that the patient understands instructions for an MRI when the patient makes which statement?
    1. "I will have a small Band-Aid on the puncture site."
    2. "I will need to wash my hair following the MRI."
    3. "I should avoid eating or drinking for 4 hours after the procedure."
    4. "I should be sure to remove all metal jewelry."

12. The nurse is providing care for a patient scheduled for a computerized tomography (CT) scan of the brain. Which of the following statements should be included in the patient teaching? **Select all that apply.**
    1. "You will need to lie still for 1 to 2 hours during the exam."
    2. "Notify the staff if you have any nausea, sweating, or itching during the exam."
    3. "Mild sedation can be given if you become uncomfortable."
    4. "You may have a feeling of warmth throughout your body after the dye is injected."
    5. "The table may be moved to various positions during the test."
    6. "This test can't be used if you have any metal in your body."

Nursing Care of Patients With Central Nervous System Disorders

48

VOCABULARY

Match the term with the correct definition.

1. _____ Contralateral hemiparesis
2. _____ Ipsilateral hemiplegia
3. _____ Quadriplegia
4. _____ Paraplegia
5. _____ Photophobia
6. _____ Bradykinesia
7. _____ Craniotomy
8. _____ Encephalitis
9. _____ Nuchal rigidity
10. _____ Prodromal

1. All four extremities paralyzed
2. Sensitive to light
3. Inflammation of the brain
4. Slow movement
5. Surgical opening in the skull
6. Paralyzed on same side
7. Paralyzed lower extremities
8. Neck pain and stiffness
9. Weak on opposite side
10. Warning sign

DRUGS USED FOR CENTRAL NERVOUS SYSTEM DISORDERS

Match the drug with its action.

1. _____ Mannitol
2. _____ Tacrine (Cognex)
3. _____ Carbamazepine (Tegretol)
4. _____ Dexamethasone (Decadron)
5. _____ Levodopa/carbidopa (Sinemet)

1. Anticonvulsant
2. Osmotic diuretic
3. Cholinesterase inhibitor
4. Converts to dopamine in the brain
5. Corticosteroid

ALZHEIMER'S DISEASE REVIEW

Match the stage of disease with its primary symptom.

1. _____ Stage 1
2. _____ Stage 2
3. _____ Stage 3
4. _____ Stage 4

1. Terminal
2. Confused
3. Forgetful
4. Ambulatory dementia

CENTRAL NERVOUS SYSTEM DISORDERS

Match the signs and symptoms at the left with the correct disorders at the right.

1. _____ Unconscious at accident scene
2. _____ Polyuria and polydipsia following head injury
3. _____ Hypotension, loss of sympathetic function
4. _____ Nuchal rigidity
5. _____ High blood pressure, bradycardia, diaphoresis
6. _____ Brief period of staring
7. _____ Automatic repetitive movement such as picking or lip smacking
8. _____ Status epilepticus
9. _____ Cushing's triad
10. _____ Cerebral vasoconstriction followed by vasodilation

1. Spinal shock
2. Absence seizure
3. Migraine
4. Increased intracranial pressure (ICP)
5. Meningitis
6. Diabetes insipidus
7. Autonomic dysreflexia
8. Complex partial seizure
9. Epidural bleed
10. Continuous seizure

SPINAL DISORDERS

Determine whether each of the following symptoms is associated with lumbar spine or cervical spine dysfunction. Indicate L for lumbar and C for cervical.

1. _____ Radiating pain to the ankle
2. _____ Deltoid weakness
3. _____ Diminished triceps reflex
4. _____ Footdrop
5. _____ Inability to walk on the toes

CRITICAL THINKING: SPINAL CORD INJURY

Mr. Granger is a 23-year-old admitted to your unit with a C5–C6 spinal cord injury after an automobile accident. You collect the following data:

Subjective Data

Pain in cervical spine
No sensation below the level of the injury

Objective Data

No movement below the level of the injury
Blood pressure 80/60 mm Hg
Pulse 45 beats per minute
Respirations shallow
Temperature 97°F (36.1°C)

1. Explain Mr. Granger's hypotension, hypothermia, and bradycardia. _____
_____
_____

2. Why are Mr. Granger's respirations shallow? _____
_____
_____
_____

3. Explain the purpose of each of the following therapies. How will they benefit Mr. Granger?
   a. Cervical traction: _____
   _____
   _____
   _____

   b. Vasopressor administration: _____
   _____
   _____
   _____

   c. Insertion of a urinary catheter: _____
   _____
   _____
   _____

4. Mr. Granger suddenly becomes anxious and dyspneic. He is using his accessory muscles with each breath. Explain what might be happening. _____
_____
_____
_____
_____

5. What treatment would you expect for the dyspnea, and why will it be beneficial to Mr. Granger? _____

_____

_____

_____

6. List two priority nursing diagnoses and goals for the acute stage of Mr. Granger's injury. _____

_____

_____

_____

_____

7. What are two health learning needs Mr. Granger faces in his acute stage? _____

_____

_____

_____

REVIEW QUESTIONS—CONTENT REVIEW

Choose the best answer unless directed otherwise.

1. Which of the following settings is most therapeutic for an agitated patient with a head injury?
   1. A day room with family visitors and a variety of caregivers
   2. A semiprivate room with one or two consistent caregivers
   3. A ward with other patients who have head injuries and volunteers to assist with needs
   4. A hallway near the nurse's station with adequate sensory stimulation

2. Decreasing level of consciousness is a symptom of which of the following physiological phenomena?
   1. Increased ICP
   2. Sympathetic response
   3. Parasympathetic response
   4. Increased cerebral blood flow

3. Which of the following blood pressure changes alerts the nurse to increasing ICP and should be reported immediately?
   1. Gradual increase
   2. Rapid drop followed by gradual increase
   3. Widening pulse pressure
   4. Rapid fluctuations

4. Which of the following nursing interventions will help prevent a further increase in ICP?
   1. Encourage fluids.
   2. Elevate the head of the bed.
   3. Provide physical therapy.
   4. Reposition the patient frequently.

REVIEW QUESTIONS—TEST PREPARATION

Choose the best answer unless directed otherwise.

5. A 90-year-old nursing home resident with stage 2 Alzheimer's disease is found alone and crying in the dining room. She says she lost her mother and doesn't know what to do. Which response by the nurse will help calm the resident?
   1. "Remember your mother has been dead for 30 years. You forgot again, didn't you?"
   2. "I'm sorry you lost your mother; let's go and try to find her."
   3. "Are you feeling frightened? I'm here and I will help you."
   4. "You are 90 years old. It is impossible for your mother to still be living. I know if you try, you can figure out what to do."

6. A patient asks the nurse what side effects to expect from a muscle relaxant medication that has been prescribed. Which of the following side effects should the nurse relate?
   1. Hypoglycemia
   2. Hypotension
   3. Drowsiness
   4. Dyspnea

7. A nurse caring for a patient with a herniated lumbar disk develops a plan of care for impaired mobility related to nerve compression. Which patient outcome indicates that the plan has been successful?
   1. The patient rates the pain at 3 to 4 on a 0-to-10 scale.
   2. The patient has full range of motion of the upper extremities.
   3. The patient demonstrates correct self-administration of analgesics.
   4. The patient is able to ambulate 25 feet without pain.

8. Which of the following problems during the immediate postoperative course following lumbar microdiskectomy should be reported to the physician immediately?
   1. Incisional pain
   2. Two-inch area of bleeding on dressing
   3. Inability to move affected leg
   4. Muscle spasm of affected leg

9. A patient with a brain tumor is admitted to the medical unit to begin radiation treatments. Which nursing action should take priority?
   1. Pad the patient's side rails.
   2. Assess the patient's pain level.
   3. Teach the patient what to expect during radiation treatments.
   4. Place the patient in isolation.

10. Which nursing interventions can help prevent falls in a patient with Parkinson's disease? **Select all that apply.**
    1. Keep the patient's call light within reach.
    2. Apply a soft vest restraint when the patient is in bed.
    3. Avoid use of throw rugs.
    4. Maintain the patient's bed in a low position.
    5. Encourage the patient to be independent for as long as possible.
    6. Provide a cane or walker for ambulation.

11. The nurse is counseling a young woman with a spinal cord injury at C7. Which of the following birth control options would the nurse recommend for this client? Select all that apply.
    1. Condom
    2. Oral contraceptives
    3. Diaphragm
    4. Implantable device
    5. Intrauterine device
    6. No birth control is needed because she will be infertile.

Nursing Care of Patients With Cerebrovascular Disorders

49

VOCABULARY

Match the term with the correct definition.

1. _____ Thrombotic
2. _____ Aphasia
3. _____ Dysphagia
4. _____ Hemianopsia
5. _____ Flaccid
6. _____ Ataxia
7. _____ Diplopia
8. _____ Hemiplegia
9. _____ Penumbra
10. _____ Ischemic

1. Difficulty swallowing
2. Deficient blood flow to organ or tissue
3. Inability to speak or understand language
4. Vision lost in half of visual field
5. Without muscle tone
6. Imbalanced, staggering gait
7. Caused by a clot
8. Healthy tissue surrounding an infarct
9. Double vision
10. Paralyzed on one side of the body

DRUGS USED FOR CEREBROVASCULAR DISORDERS

Match the drug with its action.

1. _____ Heparin
2. _____ Clopidogrel (Plavix)
3. _____ Tissue plasminogen activator (tPA)
4. _____ Simvastatin (Zocor)

1. Anticoagulant
2. Cholesterol-lowering agent
3. Antiplatelet
4. Thrombolytic

CRITICAL THINKING: STROKE

Read the following case study and answer the questions.

Mrs. Saunders is a 70-year-old retired secretary admitted to your unit from the emergency department with a diagnosis of stroke (cerebrovascular accident, or CVA). She has a history of hypertension and atherosclerosis, and she had a carotid endarterectomy 6 years ago. She is 40% over her ideal body weight and has a 20-pack-year smoking history. Her daughter says her mother has been having short episodes of confusion and memory loss for the past few weeks. This morning she found her mother slumped to the right in her recliner, unable to speak.

1. Explain the pathophysiology of a CVA. Which type of stroke is most likely the cause of Mrs. Saunders's symptoms? _____

_____

_____

_____

2. Mrs. Saunders is flaccid on her right side. What is the term used to describe this? _____

_____

_____

3. Which hemisphere of Mrs. Saunders' brain is damaged?

_____

_____

_____

4. List four risk factors for stroke evident in Mrs. Saunders's history. _____

_____

_____

_____

5. Mrs. Saunders appears to understand when you speak to her but is only able to speak in garbled words. What is the term for this? _____

_____

_____

6. Neurologic checks are ordered every 2 hours for 4 hours, then every 4 hours for 4 days. When you enter her room and call her name, she opens her eyes. She is able to squeeze your hand with her left hand. However, she is only able to make incomprehensible sounds. What is her score on the Glasgow Coma Scale? _____

_____

7. List at least three early symptoms of increasing intracranial pressure (ICP) for which you will be vigilant. (You may want to refer back to Chapter 48.)

_____

_____

_____

_____

8. List two medications that the physician may order. Why might they be used? _____

_____

_____

_____

9. Identify a nursing diagnosis related to Mrs. Saunders's right-sided paralysis. List three interventions to prevent complications. _____

_____

_____

_____

10. How will you protect Mrs. Saunders's skin? List at least three interventions. _____

_____

_____

_____

11. As you enter Mrs. Saunders's room on her third day on your unit, you find her agitated, trying to speak, and trying to get out of bed. List at least three ways to try to find out what she wants. _____

_____

_____

_____

12. What should you do before feeding Mrs. Saunders for the first time? _____

_____

_____

_____

13. Mrs. Saunders has some difficulty swallowing and pockets her food in her right cheek. List three interventions you can try. _____

_____

_____

_____

14. Mrs. Saunders begins to move her right hand slightly and is able to say her daughter's name when she enters the room. She is prepared for discharge to a rehabilitation facility. List three ways you can prepare her family for her move and her eventual discharge home.

_____

_____

_____

_____

15. What class of drugs might be ordered for Mrs. Saunders to prevent another stroke?

_____

_____

_____

REVIW QUESTIONS—CONTENT REVIEW

Choose the best answer unless directed otherwise.

1. What is the term or acronym for a temporary impairment of cerebral circulation that causes symptoms lasting minutes to hours but results in no permanent neurologic changes?
   1. TIA
   2. CVA
   3. SAH
   4. Stroke

2. A post–myocardial infarction (MI) patient experiencing atrial fibrillation is most at risk for which type of stroke?
   1. Hemorrhagic stroke
   2. Embolic stroke
   3. Thrombotic stroke
   4. Cerebral aneurysm

REVIEW QUESTIONS—TEST PREPARATION

Choose the best answer unless directed otherwise.

3. A nurse approaches a hospitalized poststroke patient from the patient's left side to provide morning care. The patient is staring straight ahead and does not respond to the nurse's presence or voice. Which action should the nurse take first?
   1. Walk to the other side of the bed and try again.
   2. Speak more loudly and clearly.
   3. Wave his or her fingers in front of the patient's face.
   4. Use a picture board to explain to the patient what the nurse is going to do.

4. A 72-year-old man is admitted to a skilled care facility following a stroke. When the nursing assistant is bathing him, he makes a sexual remark and tries to touch her inappropriately. The assistant finishes the bath, then tells the licensed practical nurse (LPN) in charge, "I refuse to take care of that dirty old man!" Which response by the nurse is best?
   1. "The next time he tries to touch you inappropriately, lightly smack his hand and tell him NO!"
   2. "His stroke has made him less inhibited. We'll see if we can find a male assistant to help him."
   3. "We have to take care of all patients equally, even the dirty old men."
   4. "He didn't mean anything by it; just ignore it."

5. A patient is having difficulty swallowing following a stroke, and a swallowing evaluation is ordered. Which nursing interventions might be recommended to help prevent aspiration during eating? **Select all that apply.**
   1. Place the patient in a semi-Fowler's position.
   2. Encourage the use of a straw for liquids.
   3. Provide clear liquids only until the patient can swallow solid foods.
   4. Have the patient swallow twice after each bite.
   5. Place food on the unaffected side of the patient's mouth.
   6. Check the patient's mouth for pocketing of food.

6. A patient is unable to control his bowels after a subarachnoid hemorrhage. Which intervention by the nurse can help reduce episodes of bowel incontinence?
   1. Ask the patient frequently if he has to have a bowel movement.
   2. Place incontinence pads on the patient's bed and chair.
   3. Toilet the patient according to his preillness schedule, whether or not he feels the urge.
   4. Take care not to embarrass the patient when incontinent episodes occur.

7. The nurse needs to administer aspirin 62 mg to a poststroke patient. It is supplied in 1-grain tablets. How many tablets should the nurse prepare? _____

8. A patient is hospitalized following a stroke. Three days after admission, the patient is able to converse clearly with the nurse in the morning. Early in the afternoon, the patient's daughter runs out of the room and says, "My mother can't talk. Somebody help!" Which response by the nurse is best?
   1. Explain to the daughter that this is not uncommon, especially in the afternoon when the patient is tired from morning care activities.
   2. Do a quick assessment to confirm the change in the patient's status, then notify the registered nurse (RN) or physician stat.
   3. Call the speech therapist to come and do a comprehensive speech assessment.
   4. Show the daughter how to help her mother do the speech exercises that were provided by the therapist.

9. The nurse is caring for a patient recently admitted with a CVA. The patient is experiencing nausea and begins to vomit. Which of the following actions should the nurse take first?
   1. Call for an aide to get suction set up.
   2. Assist the patient to turn to his side.
   3. Give an antiemetic as ordered.
   4. Perform a test for blood on the emesis.

10. The nurse is providing care for a patient with a hemorrhagic stroke. Which of the following medication orders would the nurse question? **Select all that apply.**
    1. Simvastatin (Zocor)
    2. Clopidogrel (Plavix)
    3. Carbamazepine (Tegretol)
    4. Tissue plasminogen activator (tPA)
    5. Metoprolol (Toprol)
    6. Warfarin (Coumadin)

11. A 67-year-old gentleman being evaluated and treated in the emergency department for a CVA has clopidogrel (Plavix) ordered per os (PO) now. Which of the following would cause the nurse to hold the medication? **Select all that apply.**
    1. The patient has weak grip strength in the right hand and strong in the left.
    2. The patient's smile is crooked.
    3. The patient's gag reflex is positive.
    4. The patient's voice sounds gurgly after taking a sip of water.
    5. The patient's blood pressure is 168/90 mm Hg.
    6. The patient has an allergy to aspirin.

Nursing Care of Patients With Peripheral Nervous System Disorders

50

VOCABULARY

Fill in the blanks with the correct terms.

1. Muscles that are not used become wasted, or _____.

2. Some diseases are characterized by remissions and _____.

3. Nerve pain is also called _____.

4. An early symptom of myasthenia gravis is drooping eyelids, also called _____.

5. Symptoms of Guillain-Barré syndrome are caused by _____ of axons.

6. Myasthenia gravis is sometimes treated with _____, which separates blood cells from plasma to remove antibodies.

7. Muscle twitching, or _____, occur in amyotrophic lateral sclerosis.

8. Medications for myasthenia gravis that can increase acetylcholine at the neuromuscular junction are called _____ agents.

PERIPHERAL NERVOUS SYSTEM DISORDERS

Underline incorrect information in the following case studies. Write the correct information in the space provided.

1. Ms. Mary Garvey sees her physician because she has been seeing double off and on for several weeks and has been fatigued. Her physician suspects myasthenia gravis and schedules her for a carotid ultrasound. He confirms his suspicions with a Tensilon (edrophonium chloride) test. He explains to Ms. Garvey that she has a disease that is characterized by a decrease in the neurotransmitter norepinephrine. He begins her on Mastodon and prednisone. Her nurse teaches her the importance of getting regular exercise and recommends joining a local health and exercise club. _____ _____ _____

2. Mr. Tom Newby has a history of trigeminal neuralgia. He enters the emergency department with severe pain in his left wrist. The physician orders a narcotic analgesic because Mr. Newby's third cranial nerve is inflamed. Once the acute pain has subsided, Mr. Newby is discharged with instructions to get plenty of fresh air and to take his gabapentin (Neurontin) as ordered. _____ _____ _____

3. Mrs. Mattie Schultz is admitted with exacerbated multiple sclerosis (MS). Her legs are becoming weaker, causing difficulty walking, and she has been having difficulty swallowing. You know that build up of myelin on her neurons is responsible for her weakness. You assess her for stressors that might have caused her exacerbation, such as a urinary tract infection (UTI) or upper respiratory tract infection (URI). Mrs. Schultz is started on thyroid-stimulating hormone (TSH) to stimulate her thyroid, which will help reduce her symptoms. She is also placed on trimethoprim/sulfamethoxazole (Bactrim)

for the UTI you identified through your excellent assessment and on diazepam (Valium) for urinary retention.

_____

_____

_____

_____

CRITICAL THINKING

Read the following case study and answer the questions.

Reverend Wilson is a 50-year-old minister who sees his physician when he develops weakness in his arms and legs and has difficulty carrying out his job duties. He is diagnosed with amyotrophic lateral sclerosis (ALS).

1. Reverend Wilson's wife asks what ALS is. How do you describe it for her? _____

_____

_____

2. Reverend Wilson returns to the physician's office several months after his initial diagnosis because he fell walking to the podium to preach. What is happening? What can he do about it? _____

_____

_____

3. Reverend Wilson is concerned about continuing in his job and asks if his mind is going to be affected. How do you respond? _____

_____

_____

4. He develops painful muscle spasms. What medications might be ordered to help relieve them? _____

_____

_____

5. Reverend Wilson stabilizes for a while. A year later, he is admitted to the hospital with aspiration pneumonia. What probably happened? What nursing diagnosis is appropriate in this situation? List an appropriate goal and two or three interventions. _____

_____

_____

_____

_____

6. Reverend Wilson's condition deteriorates, and he has to retire. He becomes confined to a wheelchair. He has a gastrostomy tube inserted because he is no longer able to swallow. What additional nursing diagnoses are now appropriate? _____

_____

_____

REVIEW QUESTIONS—CONTENT REVIEW

Choose the best answer unless directed otherwise.

1. Which drug class is used to reduce symptoms of muscle weakness from myasthenia gravis?
   1. Anticholinesterase drugs
   2. Anticholinergic drugs
   3. Adrenergic drugs
   4. Beta-blocker drugs

2. Which of the following nursing interventions will help prevent complications in the patient with Bell's palsy?
   1. Megavitamin therapy
   2. Elastic bandages
   3. Application of ice to the affected area
   4. Lubricating eye drops

3. Which data collection activity will help the nurse determine if the patient with Bell's palsy is receiving adequate nutrition?
   1. Monitor meal trays.
   2. Measure intake and output.
   3. Check twice-weekly weights.
   4. Evaluate swallowing reflex.

REVIEW QUESTIONS—TEST PREPARATION

Choose the best answer unless directed otherwise.

4. A 32-year-old patient is admitted to a medical unit with a diagnosis of Guillain-Barré syndrome. The patient's legs are weak, causing difficulty walking without assistance. Which of the following is most likely responsible for this syndrome?
   1. Bacterial infection
   2. Heredity
   3. High-fat diet
   4. Autoimmune reaction

5. Patients with Guillain-Barré syndrome should be closely monitored. Which of the following lab results is most important to monitor for acute complications?
   1. Blood urea nitrogen (BUN) and creatinine
   2. Arterial blood gases (ABG)
   3. Hemoglobin (Hgb) and hematocrit (Hct)
   4. Serum potassium

6. A woman sees her primary care provider because of extreme fatigue for the past 2 months; she has difficulty lifting even light objects. Her physician suspects myasthenia gravis. Which of the following tests should the nurse anticipate assisting with to confirm this diagnosis?
   1. Mestinon test
   2. Quinine tolerance test
   3. Pulmonary function studies
   4. Tensilon test

7. A 39-year-old patient sees the physician after falling twice for seemingly no reason. Diagnostic tests are done, and the patient is diagnosed with MS. Which of the following explanations will help the patient understand the disease?
   1. "You have a buildup of myelin in your nervous system, causing congestion and muscle weakness."
   2. "You are missing a neurotransmitter that is important to muscle contraction."
   3. "The receptor sites on your muscles are damaged, so they can't contract correctly."
   4. "The insulation on your nerve cells is damaged, which slows the impulses to the muscles."

8. A patient who is newly diagnosed with MS asks what medications are used to help control symptoms and treat the disease. Which of the following medications would the nurse include in the teaching?
   1. Acyclovir (Zovirax)
   2. Adrenocorticotropic hormone (ACTH)
   3. Thyrotropin
   4. Diphenhydramine (Benadryl)

9. A home care nurse is developing a plan of care designed to prevent complications in a patient with impaired respiratory function secondary to a neurological disorder. Which of the following would the nurse include in the plan?
   1. Antibiotics as needed
   2. Elevate the head of the bed
   3. Bedrest
   4. Suction every 4 hours

10. A nurse is preparing an intramuscular injection of prednisolone acetate, 30 mg. It is supplied as 50 mg/mL. How many milliliters should the nurse prepare?

    _____

11. The nurse notes frequent muscle twitching when collecting admission data on a patient admitted for increasing muscle weakness. Which of the following terms should be used to document this?
    1. Fasciculations
    2. Atrophy
    3. Chorea
    4. Neuropathy

12. A 19-year-old student develops trigeminal neuralgia. Which of the following actions is most likely to trigger pain?
    1. Sleeping
    2. Eating
    3. Reading
    4. Cooking

Understanding the Sensory System

CHECKLIST FOR LEARNING SUCCESS

Review of Anatomy and Physiology and Aging Changes	Major Disorders	Nursing Assessment	Diagnostic Tests	Interventions	Common Medications
❑ Eye structures	❑ **Vision:**	❑ Medical history	❑ **Vision:**	❑ **Vision:**	❑ **Vision:**
❑ Eye function	❑ Eye infections/	❑ Psychosocial history	❑ Amsler grid	❑ Corrective eyewear	❑ Cycloplegics
❑ Ear structures	inflammation	❑ Medications	❑ Angiography	❑ Trabeculoplasty	❑ Cholinergics
❑ Ear function	❑ Refractive errors	❑ Physical examination	❑ Digital imaging	❑ Trabeculectomy	(miotics)
❑ Aging effects	❑ Blindness	❑ **Vision:**	❑ Intraocular pressure	❑ Cyclocryotherapy	❑ Acetazolamide
	❑ Diabetic retinopathy	❑ Pupillary reflexes	❑ Ophthalmoscopy	❑ Iridotomy/	(Diamox)
	❑ Retinal detachment	❑ Accommodation	❑ Slit lamp	iridectomy	❑ Timolol (Timoptic)
	❑ Glaucoma	❑ Romberg's test	❑ Visual acuity	❑ Scleral buckling	❑ **Hearing:**
	❑ Cataracts	❑ **Hearing:**	❑ **Hearing:**	❑ Supportive services	❑ Cerumenolytics
	❑ Macular	❑ Rinne test	❑ Audiometric	❑ Postoperative eye	
	degeneration	❑ Weber test	❑ Caloric test	care	
	❑ **Hearing:**		❑ Otoscopic	❑ Irrigation	
	❑ Hearing loss		❑ Tympanometry	❑ **Hearing:**	
	❑ Infection			❑ Hearing aids	
	❑ Otosclerosis			❑ Myringotomy	
	❑ Ménière's disease			❑ Stapedectomy	
				❑ Postoperative	
				ear care	

51

Sensory System Function, Assessment, and Therapeutic Measures: Vision and Hearing

STRUCTURES OF THE EYE

Label the following structures.

Anterior chamber	Fovea	Pupil
Aqueous humor	Inferior rectus muscle	Retina
Canal of Schlemm	Iris	Retinal artery and vein
Choroid layer	Lens	Sclera
Ciliary body	Optic disc	Superior rectus muscle
Conjunctiva	Optic nerve	Suspensory ligaments
Cornea	Posterior chamber	Vitreous humor

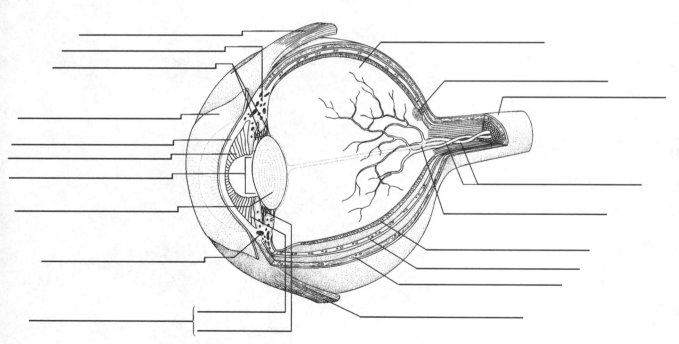

STRUCTURES OF THE EAR

Label the following structures.

Auricle   Incus
Cochlea   Malleus
Ear canal   Semicircular canals
Eighth cranial nerve   Stapes
Eustachian tube   Tympanic membrane   (eardrum)

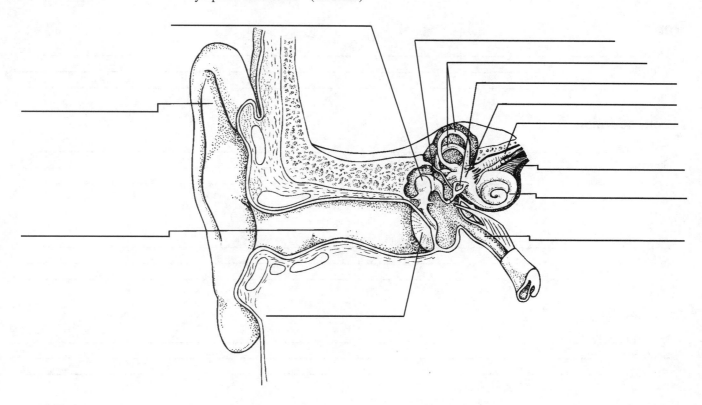

VISION

Number the following in the proper sequence as they are involved in the process of producing a visual image from the beginning to end.

_____ Cornea   _____ Occipital lobe

_____ Vitreous humor   _____ Lens

_____ Optic nerve   _____ Retina

_____ Aqueous humor

HEARING

Number the following in the order they function in the process of hearing when sound waves enter the ear canal.

_____ Eardrum   _____ Stapes

_____ Oval window   _____ Fluid in the cochlea

_____ Incus   _____ Hair cells in the organ of Corti

_____ Eighth cranial nerve _____ Temporal lobes

_____ Malleus

VOCABULARY

Define the following terms and use them in a sentence.

Nystagmus

Definition: _____

Sentence: _____

_____

Tropia

Definition: _____

Sentence: _____

_____

Accommodation

Definition: _____

Sentence: _____

_____

Ptosis

Definition: _____

Sentence: _____

_____

Arcus senilis

Definition: _____

Sentence: _____

_____

Ophthalmologist

Definition: _____

Sentence: _____

_____

Optometrist

Definition: _____

Sentence: _____

_____

Optician

Definition: _____

Sentence: _____

_____

DIAGNOSTIC TESTS

Fill in the table.

Assessment Test	Purpose of Test	Normal Test Results
Snellen chart	_____	OD 20/20, OS 20/20, OU 20/20
Visual fields	_____	_____
Cardinal fields of gaze	Extraocular movement	
Accommodation	_____	Eyes turn inward and pupils constrict when focusing on a near object. Air conduction greater than bone conduction.
Rinne	_____	
Weber	_____	_____
Romberg's	Balance/vestibular function	_____

CRITICAL THINKING

Read the following case study and answer the questions.

Ms. Sally Litley works on a computer as a data processor. She reports that she has recurring eye discomfort about 2 hours after she begins work each day.

1. What might the nurse suspect is occurring with Ms. Litley? _____

_____

_____

2. For what environmental factors should the nurse gather data? _____

_____

_____

3. To protect Ms. Litley from eye strain, what safety measures should be implemented in her office? _____

_____

_____

REVIEW QUESTIONS—CONTENT REVIEW

Choose the best answer unless directed otherwise.

1. Which of the following, if documented in the patient's history, would indicate that the patient has a normal corneal light reflex?
   1. The eye focuses the image in the center of the pupil.
   2. The eyes converge to focus on the light.
   3. Constriction of both pupils occurs in response to bright light.
   4. Light is reflected at the same spot in both eyes.

2. When testing visual fields, the nurse examines which of the following parts of vision?
   1. Peripheral vision
   2. Near vision
   3. Distance vision
   4. Central vision

3. Which of the following terms would indicate to the nurse that a substance is toxic to the ear?
   1. Otoplasty
   2. Otalgia
   3. Ototoxic
   4. Tinnitus

4. Which of the following tests would the nurse use as an initial screening test to determine hearing loss?
   1. Romberg's test
   2. Otoscopic examination
   3. Caloric test
   4. Whisper voice test

5. Which of the following would the nurse use to document a finding that the patient's ear is draining?
   1. Otorrhea
   2. Otalgia
   3. Ototoxic
   4. Tinnitus

6. The nurse is reading the patient's medical history. Which of the following terms indicates that the patient has a hearing loss caused by aging?
   1. Otoplasty
   2. Otalgia
   3. Presbycusis
   4. Tinnitus

REVIEW QUESTIONS—TEST PREPARATION

Choose the best answer unless directed otherwise.

7. Which of the following explanations would the nurse give to the patient who had a Snellen chart finding of 20/80?
   1. "You can see at 80 feet what those with normal vision can see at 20 feet."
   2. "You can see at 20 feet what those with normal vision can see at 80 feet."
   3. "You can see four times farther than those with normal vision can see."
   4. "Your vision is normal."

8. The examiner shines a light in the patient's eyes and notes that the pupils are round and constrict from 4 to 2 mm bilaterally. Next, the examiner asks the patient to focus on a far object, then on the examiner's finger as it is brought from a distance of 3 feet to 5 inches. The pupils constrict bilaterally and the eyes turn inward. Which of the following would be the correct documentation of these findings?
   1. Pupils 2 mm.
   2. Pupils constricted.
   3. Pupils equal, round, and reactive to light and accommodation (PERRLA).
   4. Pupils normal.

9. In planning safe care for the older adult, which of the following conditions does the nurse recognize would cause visual problems? **Select all that apply.**
   1. Glaucoma
   2. Cataracts
   3. Arcus senilis
   4. Macular degeneration
   5. Esotropia
   6. Presbycusis

10. Which of the following statements does the nurse understand is true concerning air conduction of sound in the ear?
    1. It is caused by the vibration of bones in the skull.
    2. It is less efficient than bone conduction.
    3. It is heard longer than bone conduction.
    4. It is caused by transmission of heat through the air.

11. Which of the following data collection findings could indicate to the nurse that the patient has a hearing loss? **Select all that apply.**
    1. Patient converses easily with nurse.
    2. Patient answers questions appropriately.
    3. Patient's face is relaxed during conversation.
    4. Patient speaks in a very loud voice.
    5. Patient turns toward person speaking.
    6. Patient is withdrawn.

12. Which of the following statements would the nurse understand is true when checking normal auditory acuity using the Rinne test?
    1. The patient perceives sound equally in both ears.
    2. Air conduction is heard longer than bone conduction in both ears.
    3. Bone conduction is heard longer than air conduction in both ears.
    4. The patient's left ear will perceive the sound better than the right ear.

13. Which of the following subjective data questions would assist the nurse in assessing the patient's eye health?
    1. "Have you had any recent upper respiratory infections?"
    2. "Have you ridden in a car recently?"
    3. "Have you been scuba diving lately?"
    4. "Have you seen halos around lights?"

14. When assessing the external ear, the nurse palpates a small protrusion of the helix called a Darwin tubercle. The nurse would document this finding as which of the following?
    1. A normal finding
    2. An abnormal finding
    3. A normal finding only in the older adult
    4. An abnormal finding only in the older adult

Nursing Care of Patients With Sensory Disorders: Vision and Hearing

52

VOCABULARY

Match the following terms with their appropriate definitions.

1. _____ Carbuncle
2. _____ Cholesteatoma
3. _____ Mastoiditis
4. _____ Barotrauma
5. _____ Labyrinthitis
6. _____ Presbycusis

1. Hearing loss caused by aging
2. Inflammation or infection of the inner ear
3. Complication of otitis media
4. Epithelial cystlike sac filled with skin and sebaceous material
5. Several hair follicles forming an abscess
6. Pressure in the middle ear caused by atmospheric changes

ERRORS OF REFRACTION

Draw pictures showing the eye size and focal point differences in (a) hyperopia and (b) myopia.

PRESBYOPIA

Circle the seven errors in the following paragraph and insert the correct information.

Presbyopia is a condition in which the lenses increase their elasticity resulting in a decrease in ability to focus on far objects. The loss of elasticity causes light rays to focus in front of the retina, resulting in hyperopia. This condition is usually associated with aging and generally occurs before age 40. Because accommodation for close vision is accomplished by lens contraction, people with presbyopia exhibit the ability to see objects at close range. They often compensate for blurred close vision by holding objects to be viewed closer. Complaints of eye strain and mild occipital headache are common.

VISUAL AND HEARING DATA COLLECTION

Describe how the nurse would know that a patient has the following condition based on data collection (include diagnostic tests and examinations).

Macular degeneration (dry type) _____

_____

Cataract _____

_____

Hordeolum _____

_____

Acute angle-closure glaucoma _____

_____

External otitis _____

_____

Impacted cerumen _____

_____

Otitis media _____

_____

Otosclerosis _____

GLAUCOMA

Circle the seven errors in the following paragraph and insert the correct information.

Glaucoma may be characterized by abnormal pressure outside the eyeball. This pressure causes damage to the cells of the acoustic nerve, the structure responsible for transmitting visual information from the ear to the brain. The damage is evident, progressive, and reversible until the end stage, when loss of central vision occurs and eventually blindness. Once glaucoma occurs, the patient can be cured.

CONDUCTIVE HEARING LOSS

Circle the six errors in the following paragraph and insert the correct information.

Conductive hearing loss is interference with conduction of light waves through the external auditory canal, eardrum, or middle ear. The inner ear is involved in a pure conductive hearing loss. Conductive hearing loss is a neural problem. Causes of conductive hearing loss include cerumen, foreign bodies, infection, perforation of the tympanic membrane, trauma, fluid in the middle ear, cysts, tumor, and otosclerosis. Many causes of conductive hearing loss, such as infection, foreign bodies, or impacted cerumen, cannot be corrected. Hearing devices may not improve hearing for conditions that cannot be corrected. Hearing devices are most effective with conductive hearing loss when inner ear and nerve damage are present.

OTOSCLEROSIS

Circle the nine errors in the following paragraph and insert the correct information.

Otosclerosis results from the formation of new bone along the incus. With new bone growth, the incus becomes mobile and causes conductive hearing loss. Hearing loss is most apparent after the sixth decade. Otosclerosis usually occurs less frequently in women than in men. The disease usually affects one ear. It is thought to be a hereditary disease. The primary symptom of otosclerosis is rapid hearing loss. The patient usually experiences bilateral conductive hearing loss, particularly with soft, high tones. Otectomy is the treatment of choice.

CRITICAL THINKING

Read the following case study and answer the questions.

Mr. Nyugen, age 70, reports that he has difficulty seeing at night, and has given up driving. When questioned further, he also states, "I used to be an avid reader, but I guess I'm getting too old to read. The words aren't very clear." The nurse examines his eye and finds that he is sensitive to light, has opacity of both lenses, and denies any pain.

1. What might the nurse suspect is occurring with Mr. Nyugen?

_____

_____

_____

2. For which diagnostic tests should the nurse prepare Mr. Nyugen?

_____

_____

_____

3. After the physician has made a definitive diagnosis, Mr. Nyugen asks the nurse to explain the surgical procedure for cataracts and the recovery regimen to him. Outline a teaching plan. _____

_____

_____

_____

REVIEW QUESTIONS—CONTENT REVIEW

Choose the best answer unless directed otherwise.

1. Which of the following type of eyedrops is given to constrict the pupil, permitting aqueous humor to flow around the lens?
   1. Osmotic
   2. Myotic
   3. Mydriatic
   4. Cycloplegic

2. Which of the following procedures does the nurse understand is used to correct otosclerosis?
   1. Myringotomy
   2. Myringoplasty
   3. Mastoidectomy
   4. Stapedectomy

3. The nurse understands that labyrinthitis is treated primarily with which of the following drug categories?
   1. Antihistamines
   2. Antispasmodics
   3. Anti-inflammatories
   4. Antiemetics

4. Which of the following types of hearing loss does the nurse understand is most improved with the use of a hearing aid?
   1. Conductive
   2. Sensorineural
   3. Mixed
   4. Central

5. Which of the following would the nurse teach the patient is the most common site for ear infections?
   1. Outer ear
   2. Inner ear
   3. Middle ear
   4. Semicircular canal

REVIEW QUESTIONS—TEST PREPARATION

Choose the best answer unless directed otherwise.

6. The nurse is assisting with data collection for a patient with macular degeneration. Which of the following symptoms would the nurse expect to be present? **Select all that apply.**
   1. Decreased ability to distinguish colors
   2. Sudden loss of vision
   3. Loss of near vision
   4. Loss of central vision
   5. Loss of peripheral vision
   6. Increased periodic dizziness

7. The nurse is caring for a patient after cataract surgery. Which of the following safety instructions should the nurse give this patient? **Select all that apply.**
   1. Elevate the head of your bed 45 degrees.
   2. Do not drive until after your follow-up appointment.
   3. Wear sunglasses.
   4. Avoid caffeinated beverages.
   5. Avoid straining.

8. The nurse is assisting a patient who has recently received a hearing aid. Which of the following would the nurse include in the teaching?
   1. "This device will amplify background noise so you can hear more clearly."
   2. "This occludes the ear to increase the transport of sound to nerve endings."
   3. "A hearing aid is used to amplify musical sounds."
   4. "The hearing aid improves your ability to hear."

9. The nurse is reinforcing teaching for a patient with Ménière's disease. Which of the following would the nurse explain to the patient is the triad of symptoms associated with Ménière's disease?
   1. Hearing loss, vertigo, and tinnitus
   2. Nystagmus, headache, and vomiting
   3. Nausea, vomiting, and pain
   4. Nystagmus, vomiting, and pain

10. The nurse is assisting with the plan of care for a patient with vertigo. Which of the following actions would the nurse include in the plan of care to reduce the symptoms of the patient who has vertigo?
    1. Avoid noises.
    2. Avoid sudden movements.
    3. Encourage fluid intake.
    4. Administer analgesics.

11. The nurse is caring for a patient diagnosed with acute bacterial conjunctivitis. In providing patient teaching, the nurse would tell the patient that this condition is more commonly known as which of the following?
    1. Glaucoma
    2. Astigmatism
    3. Color blindness
    4. Pinkeye

12. The nurse is collecting data on a patient with a cataract. Which of the following is usually the first symptom of a cataract that the nurse would expect a patient to report?
    1. Dry eyes
    2. Eye pain
    3. Blurring of vision
    4. Loss of peripheral vision

13. The nurse is caring for a patient after eye surgery. Which of the following nursing interventions would have the *highest* priority in the plan of care for the postoperative eye patient?
    1. Do not leave the patient unattended at any time.
    2. Teach the patient not to bend over.
    3. Report sudden onset of acute pain.
    4. Apply sandbags to either side of the head.

14. The nurse is caring for a patient with newly diagnosed glaucoma. Which of the following descriptions by the nurse would best explain glaucoma to the patient?
    1. "There is an increase in the amount of vitreous humor."
    2. "There is an increase in the intraocular pressure."
    3. "There is a decrease in the amount of aqueous humor."
    4. "There is a decrease in the intraocular pressure."

15. The nurse is caring for a patient with acute angle-closure glaucoma. Which of the following symptoms would the nurse expect to find during data collection for this patient?
    1. Flashing lights
    2. Lens opacity
    3. Halos around lights
    4. Vertigo

16. The nurse is caring for a patient after eye surgery. Which of the following activities would the nurse teach a patient to avoid so that intraocular pressure is not increased after eye surgery?
    1. Sitting upright in bed
    2. Coughing
    3. Chewing food vigorously
    4. Reading a book

unit FIFTEEN

Understanding the Integumentary System

CHECKLIST FOR LEARNING SUCCESS

Review of Anatomy and Physiology and Aging Changes	Major Disorders	Nursing Assessment	Diagnostic Tests	Interventions	Common Medications
❑ Epidermis	❑ Pressure ulcers	❑ History	❑ Cultures	❑ Debridement	❑ Antibiotics
❑ Dermis	❑ Dermatitis	❑ Color	❑ Biopsy	❑ Balneotherapy	❑ Antivirals
❑ Appendages	❑ Psoriasis	❑ Lesions	❑ Wood's light	❑ Topical medications	❑ Corticosteroids
❑ Subcutaneous tissue	❑ Herpes simplex	❑ Moisture	❑ Skin tests	❑ Dressings	❑ Analgesics
❑ Aging changes	❑ Herpes zoster	❑ Edema		❑ Negative pressure wound therapy	❑ Chemotherapy
	❑ Fungal infections	❑ Vascular markings			
	❑ Cellulitis	❑ Integrity		❑ Plastic surgery	
	❑ Acne	❑ Cleanliness		❑ Burn care	
	❑ Parasites	❑ Pressure ulcer risk assessment (Braden scale) and staging			
	❑ Pemphigus				
	❑ Malignant lesions				
	❑ Burns	❑ Burn assessment			

53 Integumentary System Function, Assessment, and Therapeutic Measures

INTEGUMENTARY STRUCTURES

Match each integumentary structure with its appropriate description.

1. _____ Epidermis
2. _____ Dermis
3. _____ Subcutaneous tissue
4. _____ Collagen fibers
5. _____ Eccrine glands
6. _____ Receptors
7. _____ Melanin
8. _____ Stratum corneum
9. _____ Stratum germinativum

1. If unbroken, prevents entry of pathogens
2. Give strength to the dermis
3. Detect changes in the external environment
4. Contains the accessory structures of the skin, such as glands
5. Made of both living and nonliving cells
6. Mitosis takes place to produce new epidermis
7. Stores fat
8. Acts as a barrier to ultraviolet (UV) light
9. Stimulated by exercise or heat

VOCABULARY

Match the word at the right with its definition at the left.

1. _____ Absence or loss of hair
2. _____ Blue-black bruise, changing to greenish-brown or yellow with time
3. _____ Diffuse redness over the skin
4. _____ Small, purplish, hemorrhagic spots on the skin
5. _____ Measure of skin elasticity and hydration

1. Ecchymosis
2. Erythema
3. Petechiae
4. Turgor
5. Alopecia

DIAGNOSTIC SKIN TESTS

Match the test with its definition.

1. _____ Skin biopsy
2. _____ Wood's light examination
3. _____ Scratch test
4. _____ Patch test

1. Superficial testing with allergen for immediate reaction
2. Excision of small piece of tissue for microscopic assessment
3. Superficial testing with allergen for delayed hypersensitivity reaction
4. Use of UV rays to detect fluorescent materials in skin and hair

PRIMARY SKIN LESIONS

Match the lesion with its description.

1. _____ Macule
2. _____ Papule
3. _____ Vesicle
4. _____ Bulla
5. _____ Pustule
6. _____ Wheal
7. _____ Plaque
8. _____ Cyst

1. Vesicle or blister larger than 1 cm
2. Flat, nonpalpable change in skin color
3. Round, transient elevation of the skin caused by dermal edema and surrounding capillary dilation
4. Patch or solid, raised lesion on the skin or mucous membrane that is greater than 1 cm
5. Palpable solid raised lesion
6. Small elevation of skin or vesicle or bulla that contains pus
7. Closed sac or pouch tumor that consists of semisolid, solid, or liquid material
8. Small raised area that contains serous fluid, less than 1 cm

CRITICAL THINKING

Read the following case study and answer the questions.

Mr. Carr is admitted to a medical unit after having a hemorrhagic stroke. His vital signs are stable, but he is disoriented except to person. He is on bed rest and is often restless. He responds appropriately to questions intermittently. His left side is flaccid, but he can move his right side. The nurse notes that Mr. Carr rarely moves himself into a different position. He is of thin build. He is receiving 5% dextrose/0.9% normal saline intravenously. He has difficulty swallowing and has not eaten. Mr. Carr is diaphoretic and his gown is damp.

1. Why is Mr. Carr at high risk for developing pressure ulcers? _____

_____

_____

_____

2. What are priority nursing diagnoses and nursing interventions for Mr. Carr related to his skin needs? _____

_____

_____

_____

REVIEW QUESTIONS—CONTENT REVIEW

Choose the best answer unless directed otherwise.

1. How do arterioles in the dermis respond to a cold environment?
   1. Dilate to release heat
   2. Constrict to release heat
   3. Dilate to conserve heat
   4. Constrict to conserve heat

2. Which of the following tissues stores fat in subcutaneous tissue?
   1. Fibrous connective tissue
   2. Stratified squamous epithelium
   3. Adipose tissue
   4. Areolar connective tissue

3. Which substances are formed when the UV rays of the sun strike the skin?
   1. Vitamin A and keratin
   2. Melanin and vitamin D
   3. Sebum and vitamin A
   4. Keratin and melanin

4. Which layer of skin, if unbroken, prevents the entry of most pathogens?
   1. Stratum corneum
   2. Papillary layer
   3. Stratum germinativum
   4. Dermis

5. White blood cells, which destroy pathogens that enter breaks in the skin, are found in which of the following structures?
   1. Stratum corneum
   2. Keratinized layer
   3. Subcutaneous tissue
   4. Adipose cells

REVIEW QUESTIONS—TEST PREPARATION

Choose the best answer unless directed otherwise.

6. The nurse is reviewing a patient chart and notes the following: "poor elasticity and dry thin skin noted." The nurse recognizes this is a normal finding for which of the following patient groups?
   1. Adolescents
   2. Young adults
   3. Middle-aged adults
   4. Older adults

7. When assessing a patient in hospice who is near death, the nurse notes a bluish discoloration and mottled appearance to the patient's feet and lower legs. Which of the following terms would the nurse use to best document this finding?
   1. Cyanosis
   2. Erythema
   3. Jaundice
   4. Pallor

8. A nurse is providing care for an older adult patient who reports being sensitive to cold temperatures. The nurse would base teaching on which of the following principles?
   1. There is slower cell division in the epidermis with aging.
   2. Older adults experience deterioration of collagen and elastin fibers.
   3. There is less fat in the subcutaneous layer with age.
   4. Death of melanocytes in the skin occurs with age.

9. Which of the following dressing types is most appropriate for the nurse to apply to a skin tear in an older adult patient?
   1. Moist sterile gauze
   2. OpSite transparent dressing
   3. Paste
   4. Nonadherent dressing

10. Which of the following actions should the nurse take when new petechiae are observed on a patient's skin?
    1. Cleanse the skin.
    2. Apply cool compresses.
    3. Inform the registered nurse or physician.
    4. Apply heat to the area.

11. A nurse is preparing to collect a wound culture. Which of the following would be included in the collection process? **Select all that apply.**
    1. Swab wound and wound edges in a rotating motion.
    2. Swab over areas of eschar.
    3. Use sterile saline to remove excess debris before culture.
    4. Use clean cotton-tipped swab to collect purulent drainage.
    5. Swab wound 10 times in a diagonal pattern.
    6. Obtain sterile calcium alginate swab for culture collection.

Nursing Care of Patients With Skin Disorders

54

VOCABULARY

Match the word with its definition.

1. _____ To lose color
2. _____ Inflammation of cellular or connective tissue
3. _____ Skin lesion that occurs in acne vulgaris
4. _____ Inflammation of the skin
5. _____ A fungal infection of the skin
6. _____ The growth of skin over a wound
7. _____ Thickened or hardened from continued irritation
8. _____ Disease of the nails due to fungus
9. _____ Infestation with lice
10. _____ Acute or chronic serious skin disease characterized by bullae on skin and mucous membranes
11. _____ Severe itching
12. _____ Chronic inflammatory skin disorder in which epidermal cells proliferate abnormally quickly
13. _____ Describes fluid that contains pus
14. _____ Any acute, inflammatory, purulent bacterial dermatitis
15. _____ Disease of the sebaceous glands marked by increase in the amount, and often alteration of the quality, of sebaceous secretion

1. Seborrhea
2. Pyoderma
3. Purulent
4. Psoriasis
5. Pruritus
6. Pemphigus
7. Pediculosis
8. Onychomycosis
9. Lichenified
10. Epithelialization
11. Dermatophytosis
12. Dermatitis
13. Comedo
14. Cellulitis
15. Blanch

BENIGN SKIN LESIONS

Match the lesion with its definition.

1. _____ Cyst
2. _____ Seborrheic keratosis
3. _____ Keloid
4. _____ Pigmented nevi
5. _____ Warts
6. _____ Hemangiomas

1. Small, common growths caused by a virus
2. Vascular tumors of dilated blood vessels
3. Saclike growth with a definite wall
4. Excessive scar formation at site of trauma or surgical incision
5. Light brown to dark brown patches, plaques, or papules that occur mainly in older patients
6. Flesh-colored to dark brown macule or papule

PLASTIC SURGERY PROCEDURES

Fill in the blanks.

1. A _____ is done to correct nasal shape or septal defects.
2. A _____ is referred to as a rhytidoplasty.
3. Removal of bags under the eyes is known as _____.

CRITICAL THINKING

Read the following case study and answer the questions.

Mrs. Miller, age 59, is admitted for a femoral-popliteal bypass graft. She has type 2 diabetes mellitus. After surgery, she is in the intensive care unit (ICU) and is hypotensive for 24 hours. Her operative leg is painful and she barely moves. During her bath, the nurse notes a shallow, open, reddened area 2 inches in diameter on her sacral area and a large tender purple area with intact skin on the heel of her right foot.

1. Why did these areas develop? _____
   _____
   _____

2. To plan Mrs. Miller's care, how would you stage these lesions? _____
   _____
   _____
   _____

The surgeon is notified of these areas and orders turning every 2 hours, elevation of the right foot, and a special pressure-reducing bed.

3. What is the benefit and effectiveness of each of these ordered interventions? _____
   _____
   _____
   _____

REVIEW QUESTIONS—CONTENT REVIEW

Choose the best answer unless directed otherwise.

1. Which of the following activities creates a mechanical force that can lead to the formation of a pressure ulcer?
   1. Massaging nonreddened areas
   2. Whirlpool baths
   3. Pulling a patient up in bed
   4. Range-of-motion exercises

2. Which of the following dressings should a nurse choose for a deep pressure ulcer that has purulent drainage?
   1. Sterile gauze
   2. Transparent film (OpSite)
   3. Hydrocolloid (DuoDERM)
   4. Occlusive

REVIEW QUESTIONS—TEST PREPARATION

Choose the best answer unless directed otherwise.

3. A nurse is caring for a nursing home resident with a red, pruritic skin rash. The patient is confused and scratches the rash, which results in broken skin. Which interventions will help the rash heal? **Select all that apply.**
   1. Pat the skin dry after bathing.
   2. Leave topical agent as ordered at the bedside so the patient can apply when itching is severe.
   3. Place a transparent dressing on the rash to prevent scratching.
   4. Place gloves or mitts on the patient.
   5. Keep the patient's fingernails short.
   6. Place wrist restraints on the patient during the night.

4. A patient has a wound draining moderate blood-tinged clear fluid. Which of the following would be an appropriate description of this drainage for the nurse to document?
   1. Purulent drainage
   2. Serosanguineous drainage
   3. Copious drainage
   4. Serous drainage

5. The nurse is providing care for a patient with a non-infected pressure ulcer. Which of the following actions is most appropriate?
   1. Flushing the wound with 45-psi pressure
   2. Gentle flushing with a needleless 30-mL syringe
   3. Gentle scrubbing with gauze and normal saline
   4. Flushing with a 30-mL syringe with an 18-gauge needle

6. A 62-year-old woman is admitted to the hospital with a lesion on her face that is a small, pearly papule. It has a rolled, waxy edge with crusting and ulceration. Which action by the nurse is best?
   1. Notify the physician.
   2. Clean the lesion.
   3. Place a gauze dressing on the lesion.
   4. Place an occlusive dressing on the lesion.

7. Place the wounds in correct order from stage I to stage IV.
   1. Skin appears abraded
   2. Skin red, intact, nonblanchable
   3. Full-thickness skin loss, muscle and bone showing
   4. Full-thickness skin loss, no muscle or bone involvement

8. A 92-year-old woman is admitted from a nursing home to the hospital for a colon resection. Four days postoperatively, she reports that her perineum is sore. It is reddened and has whitish discharge. She has been on three intravenous (IV) antibiotics. Which of the following problems does the nurse suspect?
   1. Candidiasis
   2. Psoriasis
   3. Herpes zoster
   4. Contact dermatitis

9. The nurse recognizes that which of the following individuals should be evaluated for a specialty bed that provides a pressure-relieving surface?
   1. A 46-year-old with scoliosis who has a urinary tract infection
   2. A 94-year-old with a Braden score of 15 and left arm weakness from a cardiovascular accident (CVA)
   3. An 88-year-old with foot drop who has a Foley catheter
   4. A 15-year-old with a Braden score of 9 who experiences pain with turning

55

Nursing Care of Patients With Burns

VOCABULARY

Match each phrase with the type of burn or burn term.

1. _____ Leathery skin, usually painless

2. _____ Pink to red moist skin, blisters may be present

3. _____ The growth of skin over a wound

4. _____ Removal of a slough or scab formed on skin and under-lying tissue of severely burned skin

5. _____ Epidermis and dermis involved, pain from exposed nerve endings

6. _____ Hard scab or dry crust from necrotic tissue

1. Débridement
2. Eschar
3. Epithelialization
4. Superficial burn
5. Partial-thickness deep burn
6. Full-thickness burn

CRITICAL THINKING

Read the following case study and answer the questions.

Mr. Patel is a 45-year-old patient in County General Hospital's Burn Unit. He was admitted with a 20% electrical burn over his right arm, right shoulder, right leg, and right foot. The entry wound is on his right shoulder and the exit wound is on his right foot. When you check on him at the beginning of your shift, you find his right radial pulse is diminished and his right forearm has a small spot that is beginning to change color to a whitish gray.

1. What might be causing his change in circulation? _____
   _____
   _____
   _____

2. What additional data should you collect? _____
   _____
   _____
   _____

3. What interventions are important to perform right away? _____
   _____
   _____
   _____

REVIEW QUESTIONS—CONTENT REVIEW

Choose the best answer unless directed otherwise.

1. Which cause of or type of burn is commonly associated with an inhalation injury?
   1. Electrical
   2. Flame
   3. Scald
   4. Contact

2. Which type of burn is caused by a hot liquid?
   1. Radiation
   2. Contact
   3. Scald
   4. Chemical

REVIEW QUESTIONS—TEST PREPARATION

Choose the best answer unless directed otherwise.

3. During morning report, a nurse is assigned a patient who is in stage III burn care. What care can the nurse anticipate providing during the shift?
   1. Dressing changes
   2. Débridement
   3. Pain management
   4. Exercises

4. A patient is brought to the emergency department with burns over 40% of the body from an apartment fire. Which assessment should take priority?
   1. Burn depth
   2. Percent of body surface burned
   3. Respiratory status
   4. Circulatory status

5. A home care nurse visits an 82-year-old patient. On entering the home, the nurse finds that the patient has just dropped a pot of boiling water on both legs. What action should the nurse take first?
   1. Call 911.
   2. Remove the clothing from the affected area.
   3. Place ice on the affected area.
   4. Assess the extent of the burn.

6. A patient has a burn encircling the left thigh from a motorcycle accident. When the nurse enters the room during rounds, the patient appears very anxious and reports a funny feeling in the left foot. What should the nurse do first?
   1. Check circulatory status in the foot and report changes.
   2. Explain that some numbness and tingling in the affected extremity are normal following a burn.
   3. Check the burn dressing for an increase in drainage.
   4. Determine the cause of the patient's anxiety.

7. A homebound patient is receiving intravenous (IV) antibiotics for an infected burn site. Instructions are to use gravity to infuse 100 mL over 1 hour. How many drops per minute should the nurse administer if the tubing has a drip factor of 15? _____

8. A nurse is providing care for a patient with burns across 30% of the body. Which of the following observations would cause the nurse to contact the registered nurse (RN) or physician?
   1. Urinary output of 50 mL in the past 2 hours
   2. Patient reports pain of 6/10; oral narcotic is due in 10 minutes
   3. Respiratory rate is 20 and oxygen saturation is 94%
   4. Blood sugar is 175 mg/dL

9. While caring for a 28-year-old patient newly admitted for burns received in a household fire, the nurse would be most concerned by which of the following?
   1. Hematocrit = 48%
   2. Blood pressure = 92/40 mm Hg
   3. Pulse = 96 beats per minute
   4. Respiratory rate = 22 per minute

unit SIXTEEN

Understanding Mental Health Care

CHECKLIST FOR LEARNING SUCCESS

Review of Basic Concepts
- ❑ Mental health
- ❑ Mental illness
- ❑ Etiologies of mental illness
- ❑ Spirituality and religion
- ❑ Coping

Major Disorders
- ❑ Anxiety disorders
- ❑ Mood disorders
- ❑ Somatoform disorders
- ❑ Schizophrenia
- ❑ Substance abuse disorders

Nursing Assessment
- ❑ Appearance and behavior
- ❑ Awareness and orientation
- ❑ Thinking
- ❑ Memory
- ❑ Speech
- ❑ Mood and affect
- ❑ Judgment
- ❑ Perception

Diagnostic Tests
- ❑ DSM-5
- ❑ Laboratory tests
- ❑ Computed tomographic (CT) scan
- ❑ Positron emission therapy (PET) scan

Interventions
- ❑ Therapeutic communication
- ❑ Milieu therapy
- ❑ Psychopharmacology
- ❑ Psychotherapies
- ❑ Cognitive therapies
- ❑ Counseling
- ❑ Group therapy
- ❑ Electroconvulsive therapy (ECT)
- ❑ Relaxation therapy

Common Medications
- ❑ Antipsychotics
- ❑ Antidepressants
- ❑ Antianxiety agents
- ❑ Anticonvulsant mood stabilizers
- ❑ Lithium
- ❑ Antiparkinsonism agents

56

Mental Health Function, Assessment, and Therapeutic Measures

VOCABULARY

Fill in the blanks with the correct terms.

1. _____ is the way one adapts to a stressor.

2. The ability to think rationally and process thoughts is referred to as _____ ability.

3. _____ is the use of medication to treat psychological disorders.

4. _____ therapy uses an electric current to stimulate neurotransmitters in severely depressed patients.

5. A therapeutic _____ is a structured environment that aids in treatment of mental health disorders.

6. Psychoanalytic therapy can help clarify the meaning, and therefore help the patient gain _____ into an event or feeling.

7. _____ is assessed by asking a patient questions such as "Where are you now?" and "What year is it?"

8. The outward expression of feelings is called _____.

DEFENSE MECHANISMS

Name the defense mechanism being used in each of the following statements.

1. A patient with cancer says, "I know if I take my vitamins, I'll be fine." _____

2. A student comes unprepared to class and says, "I woke up late because my instructor gave us so much work to do and I had to stay up all night, and my kids are sick and the car isn't working." _____

3. A man who always wanted to be a lawyer but was not accepted into law school says, "Lawyers are all crooked. I would never trust one." _____

4. A teen who didn't make the football team says, "I've decided to give up trying to play in sports. I'm much better at piano." _____

5. A woman who was raped says, "Why are you calling me to set up rape counseling? I was not raped and I do not need counseling." _____

6. A man who is passed over for a promotion yells at his son for a minor mistake, "You messed up again. You never do anything right." _____

7. An adolescent says to his mother, "I got a C on my project because you told me to do it all wrong." _____
_____

8. The woman who cheated on an examination turns in extra work and states, "Here is some extra work I did. I really want to learn this material." _____

9. A teen tells her date, "I'm sorry I can't go out tonight; I have to wash my hair." _____

10. The student nurse tells the instructor, "I don't think I can do that catheter. I am feeling sick to my stomach. I think I ate some bad food in the cafeteria." _____

CRITICAL THINKING

Read the following case study and answer the questions.

Mrs. Jewel is a 48-year-old woman admitted to your unit with cellulitis of her lower legs and diabetes mellitus. She has arthritis and morbid obesity. As you collect some initial data, you notice that her hair is dirty and unkempt, her clothes are dirty, and she has an unpleasant body odor. You also find that she does not appear to have a good understanding of her health or self-care needs. You decide to assess her mental status.

1. What factors related to Mrs. Jewel's appearance provide information about her mental status? How can you find out if this is unusual behavior for her? _____
_____
_____

2. Mrs. Jewel is alert. What questions can you ask to assess orientation? _____
_____
_____

3. How might you determine whether Mrs. Jewel's thought processes are intact? _____
_____
_____

4. What questions can you ask to determine Mrs. Jewel's recent and remote memory? _____
_____

5. How do you determine speech and ability to communicate? _____
_____
_____

6. You determine that Mrs. Jewel's affect is inappropriate. What does this mean? _____
_____
_____
_____

7. How can you evaluate Mrs. Jewel's judgment? _____
_____
_____
_____

8. How can perception be assessed? _____
_____
_____
_____

REVIEW QUESTIONS—CONTENT REVIEW

Choose the best answer unless directed otherwise.

1. Which behavior in a patient with a chronic physical illness alerts the nurse to possible mental health concerns?
   1. The patient prays for healing from illness.
   2. The patient reads self-help books to gain insight into his problems.
   3. The patient has developed ways to cope with chronic illness.
   4. The patient does not have any close friends.

2. Which defense mechanism is being used by the person who always seems to blame others for personal problems?
   1. Denial
   2. Projection
   3. Rationalization
   4. Transference

3. An office worker has an argument with the boss, and on arriving home, yells at the spouse and children. Which defense mechanism is being displayed?
   1. Rationalization
   2. Denial
   3. Reaction formation
   4. Displacement

REVIEW QUESTIONS—TEST PREPARATION

Choose the best answer unless directed otherwise.

4. The nurse is providing care for a patient immediately following electroconvulsive therapy. Which of the following nursing actions is most appropriate?
   1. Restrain the patient's extremities.
   2. Monitor the patient closely until he or she is oriented.
   3. Discharge the patient to home with instructions to rest.
   4. Administer oxygen at 4 L per minute.

5. The nurse is collecting admission data on a new patient with a long health history. Which of the following life events is considered a stressor?
   1. Gallbladder surgery at age 46
   2. Divorce at age 50
   3. Loss of job at age 55
   4. Whatever the patient says is stressful

6. A patient is admitted to the hospital mental health unit for behavior changes. The patient asks why a magnetic resonance imaging test (MRI) has been ordered. Which response by the nurse is best?
   1. "MRI can determine levels of important neurotransmitters, so the doctor will know how to treat your problem."
   2. "MRI is used to rule out physical problems that could be causing your symptoms."
   3. "MRI uses magnetic energy to treat certain psychiatric disorders."
   4. "MRI monitors electrical activity in the brain to help diagnose mental health problems."

7. A patient with panic disorder tells the nurse that she has a lot of job-related stress. Which response by the nurse is most therapeutic for this patient?
   1. "Can you identify some of the things in your job that are causing you to feel stressed?"
   2. "I'm really sorry you have so much job stress."
   3. "It is important to eliminate stressful situations so you can reduce your panic attacks."
   4. "You need to avoid stressful situations—it would be wise to start looking for another job."

8. A patient who quit drinking 4 months earlier is considering entering an inpatient alcohol rehabilitation program, and asks for the nurse's opinion. Which response by the nurse is best?
   1. "That is an excellent idea. I will help you start the paperwork."
   2. "Why do you think you need a rehabilitation program?"
   3. "What do you think you should do?"
   4. "You have done so well to be alcohol-free for 4 months."

9. A nurse is caring for a 36-year-old developmentally delayed patient admitted to the hospital for pneumonia. The patient becomes upset when the dinner tray is late, and cries "Mama" repeatedly. The patient's mother later says this is unusual behavior for the patient. Which of the following is the best explanation for this behavior?
   1. The patient is having a conversion reaction based on the hospitalization.
   2. The patient is likely having a side effect to a new medication.
   3. The patient is having symptoms of regression.
   4. The patient is repressing feelings about the illness.

10. A patient stands up during a morning community meeting and screams, "Get out of here right now! The demons are coming!" Which response by the nurse is best?
    1. "Why do you think the demons are coming?"
    2. "Yes, we should all leave right now."
    3. "If you have something to say, you must only say it when it is your turn to share."
    4. "I know you think the demons are coming, but there are no demons. You are safe here."

Nursing Care of Patients With Mental Health Disorders

57

VOCABULARY

Fill in the blanks with the correct terms.

1. A patient with schizophrenia who is unable to speak is experiencing _____.

2. A situation in which family members exist to enable a substance abuser is called _____.

3. An irrational fear is called a/an _____.

4. A repetitive thought or urge is called a/an _____.

5. Manic-depressive illness is more appropriately called _____ depression.

6. _____ spectrum disorder is characterized by social deficits and restricted repetitive behaviors.

7. People with _____ cannot distinguish between their reality and society's reality.

8. Abrupt withdrawal from alcohol may cause symptoms called _____ tremens.

9. _____ is the repeated compulsive use of a substance despite negative consequences.

10. _____ refers to the loss of ability to enjoy things that are usually pleasurable.

CRITICAL THINKING

Read the following case study and answer the questions.

You are caring for Mr. Joers, a 72-year-old man admitted to your surgical unit from a nursing home after he fell and broke his hip. He is scheduled for surgery this morning at 0800. During morning report, you learn that he has a history of Parkinson's disease, schizophrenia, and anxiety but that he was oriented and appropriate during admission and throughout the night. When you enter his room to check his vital signs and complete his preoperative checklist, he has a wild look in his eyes, and says, "Don't come near me! They told me what you're up to!"

1. What is your initial response to Mr. Joers? _____
   _____
   _____
   _____

2. What implications does his behavior have for surgery this morning? _____
   _____
   _____
   _____

3. What may have precipitated his worsening symptoms?
   _____
   _____
   _____
   _____

4. What actions do you need to take after your initial response to Mr. Joers? _____
   _____
   _____
   _____

5. What safety concerns do you have? _____

_____

_____

_____

REVIEW QUESTIONS—CONTENT REVIEW

Choose the best answer unless directed otherwise.

1. Which of the following responses to anxiety is a cause for concern?
   1. A student studies late into the night to prepare for a difficult examination.
   2. A woman takes deep breaths before going into the grocery store because shopping makes her nervous.
   3. A nurse has a glass of wine before a stressful night shift.
   4. A young man gets the opinions of several of his friends before asking a woman out.

2. Which of the following is the most effective treatment for alcoholism?
   1. Group support, such as Alcoholics Anonymous
   2. Drug therapy
   3. Electroconvulsive therapy
   4. Slowly reducing amount of alcohol consumption

REVIEW QUESTIONS—TEST PREPARATION

Choose the best answer unless directed otherwise.

3. A patient being treated with lorazepam (Ativan) during alcohol withdrawal becomes sleepy after the first two doses, then becomes difficult to arouse when the nurse attempts to give the third dose. Which of the following actions should the nurse take first?
   1. Hold the dose and notify the registered nurse (RN) or physician.
   2. Understand that tolerance will occur with benzodi-azepines and give the drug.
   3. Get the patient up and have him walk with assistance until he is more alert.
   4. Administer an antidote.

4. A patient calls a nurse into the room and says, "Quick, nurse, there is a dog in the corner. Please get him out. I am terrified of dogs." The nurse sees no dog in the corner. Which of the following responses is best?
   1. "You know we don't allow dogs in the hospital."
   2. "We have been through this before. You know full well that there is no dog in the corner."
   3. "I do not see a dog. Let's take a walk down to the snack room."
   4. "What kind of a dog is it? What makes you so scared of dogs?"

5. A patient is starting on lithium for bipolar disorder. Which of the following nutrients should the nurse teach about maintaining in the diet?
   1. Potassium
   2. Sodium
   3. Selenium
   4. Tyramine

6. Which of the following behaviors by a nurse may aggravate the behavior of a patient with schizophrenia?
   1. Providing written instructions on when to take medications
   2. Speaking in short, simple sentences
   3. Maintaining a structured environment
   4. Speaking quietly to other staff members when the patient is present

7. A patient has an order for carbamazepine (Tegretol) 150 mg twice daily for bipolar disorder. It is supplied as a suspension, 100 mg in 5 mL. How many milliliters should the nurse prepare? _____

8. Which statement by a patient with depression indicates that nursing interventions have been helpful?
   1. "His comment upset me, but I reminded myself that it really isn't true."
   2. "I feel so hopeless about everything, but I am glad you are a good listener."
   3. "I feel so much better now that I know how to control my husband's behavior."
   4. "I am really trying to understand why everyone is against me."

9. A patient is beginning treatment with paroxetine (Paxil) for unipolar depression, but after 10 days is still withdrawn and unable to participate in therapy. Which action by the nurse is best?
   1. Contact the ordering physician for an increase in the dose.
   2. Contact the ordering physician for an alternative antidepressant.
   3. Continue to support the patient while waiting for symptoms to subside.
   4. Encourage the patient to include St. John's wort, an herbal supplement, in the treatment regimen.

10. The licensed practical nurse (LPN) is providing care for a 28-year-old who is to begin taking phenelzine (Nardil) for depression. Which of the following statements indicates the need for further teaching?
    1. "It is very important that I not take other antidepressant medication while I'm on this drug."
    2. "If I notice any dizziness I should immediately stop taking the drug."
    3. "The bread and cereal food group is generally safe, but I will need to avoid certain foods from other food groups."
    4. "I will have to stop drinking beer or wine now that I'm taking this medication."